ABOUT
US

ABOUT US

ESSAYS FROM THE DISABILITY SERIES OF THE NEW YORK TIMES

EDITED AND INTRODUCED BY

PETER CATAPANO AND ROSEMARIE GARLAND-THOMSON

FOREWORD BY

ANDREW SOLOMON

LIVERIGHT PUBLISHING CORPORATION

A Division of W. W. Norton & Company

Independent Publishers Since 1923

For information about permission to reproduce selections from this book, write to
Permissions, Liveright Publishing Corporation, a division of W. W. Norton & Company, Inc.,
500 Fifth Avenue, New York, NY 10110

For information about special discounts for bulk purchases, please contact
W. W. Norton Special Sales at specialsales@wwnorton.com or 800-233-4830

Manufacturing by LSC Communications Harrisonburg
Book design by Chris Welch
Production manager: Lauren Abbate

Library of Congress Cataloging-in-Publication Data

Names: Catapano, Peter, editor, writer of introduction. | Garland-Thomson, Rosemarie, editor,
writer of introduction. | Solomon, Andrew, 1963– writer of foreword.
Title: About us : essays from the disability series of the New York times / edited and introduced
by Peter Catapano and Rosemarie Garland-Thomson ; foreword by Andrew Solomon.
Other titles: New York Times
Description: First edition. | New York, NY : Liveright Publishing Corporation, a division of
W. W. Norton & Company, [2019]
Identifiers: LCCN 2019026123 | ISBN 9781631495854 (hardcover) | ISBN 9781631495861 (epub)
Subjects: LCSH: People with disabilities—United States—Biography. | Chronically ill—
United States—Biography. | Sociology of disability—United States. | Chronic diseases—
Social aspects—United States.
Classification: LCC HV1552.3 .A36 2019 | DDC 362.4092/273—dc23
LC record available at https://lccn.loc.gov/2019026123

ISBN 978-1-63149-858-9 pbk.

Liveright Publishing Corporation, 500 Fifth Avenue, New York, N.Y. 10110
www.wwnorton.com

W. W. Norton & Company Ltd., 15 Carlisle Street, London W1D 3BS

1 2 3 4 5 6 7 8 9 0

CONTENTS

III. WORKING

IV. NAVIGATING

FOREWORD

The eugenics movement spearheaded by Francis Galton in England in the late Victorian period reached a culmination in the view that if you got rid of the misfits, you could breed a pure, advantaged race. The reach of the movement was reflected in the American campaigns to sterilize disabled people, supported in a 1927 Supreme Court decision in which Oliver Wendell Holmes wrote, "It is better for all the world, if instead of waiting to execute degenerate offspring for crime, or to let them starve for their imbecility, society can prevent those who are manifestly unfit from continuing their kind. Three generations of imbeciles are enough." Drawing on these sources, Hitler began his campaigns of genocide by gassing the disabled, presuming not only that they were polluting the larger population, but also that they were a group no one would miss. Genetic determinism presumed that the weak and disadvantaged passed along their weakness and disadvantage, and that a systematic campaign of eliminating all but the best and strongest could improve the lot of humanity.

There are two entwined arguments here, one about who makes disabled children, and the other about the worth of the lives of those disabled children. What sort of parents have children with disabilities? Every sort of parent. Nondisabled parents produce disabled children with startling regularity—and disabled people produce nondisabled children time and again. So that part of the argument is specious, at least when applied so specifically as Galton, Holmes and Hitler contemplated. More relevant to this collection is the modern argument that whether disability is passed along generationally or not, it has inherent worth, and the loss of it from our society would be a troubling depletion of human diversity. That is a more radical, philosophical challenge. Disabled lives are lives, and are charged with inherent dignity. Most people with disabilities don't wish they had never been born; most people with disabilities contribute to the world they inhabit; most people with disabilities both give more to and get more from life than their nondisabled peers may be inclined to guess. Some have rich lives despite their disability, but others would say they have rich lives at least in part because of their disability. Those arguments and the lives to which they pertain are the topic of this collection.

In 1968, the ethicist Joseph Fletcher wrote in The Atlantic Monthly, that esteemed journal of liberal thought, that there was "no reason to feel guilty about putting a Down syndrome baby away, whether it's 'put away' in the sense of hidden in a sanatorium or in a more responsible lethal sense. It is sad, yes. Dreadful. But it carries no guilt. True guilt arises only from an offense against a person, and a Down's is not a person." A lot of ink has been spilled covering our society's gradual embrace of women's rights, then racial rights, and most recently, gay rights. The shift in attitudes toward disability has been nearly as powerful, if less complete, but it has been much quieter. Today, no one would publish an article in the mainstream media that championed dehumanizing a group of disabled people as Joseph Fletcher did. What was once par for the course has become unthinkable.

Though utilitarian philosophers such as Peter Singer have proposed that parents should have the right to murder their disabled newborns, these views are deliberately polemical, widely protested and abhorrent to most people who encounter them. We have learned to value most people, and with that social advancement has come progress in improving their lives. Acceptance is protection. People with Down syndrome live nearly twice as long as they did in 1968, and many hold down jobs; some are writers or actors or models; some live at least semi-independently. That progress reflects an opening up of a society that no longer experiences the birth of a disabled child as an unmitigated tragedy, that no longer assigns chronic sorrow to the parents. This more accepting and celebratory point of view has some ascendency in the United States, but is a work in progress both here and globally; what constitutes an identity in one society or family may be a disability in another. The sociologist Ashton Applewhite quoted a matador who said, "The bull looks different when you're inside the ring." Disability is very different for disabled people than it looks to nondisabled people. What we wouldn't have opted into is not the same as what we'd now like to change.

It's hard to remember how strong the arguments were that women were lesser than men, that black people were lesser than white people, that gayness was a crime, a sin and a disease in search of a cure. It can be hard to recollect how many people still make these arguments, how many hated being under the thumb of an African-American president and how many abhor the idea of a female president, how many would deny basic services to gay and trans people, how many regard the disabled with polite disdain. Our society is rife with glass ceilings, and the disability ceiling has the fewest cracks in it. When I attended the 2018 annual convention of The Arc, the country's largest and oldest organization for people with intellectual and developmental disabilities, I was struck by how seldom we see in common life what I saw there: the meeting of disabled and nondisabled people as equals.

Increasingly, decisions about what kind of child to have are made prenatally, either through preimplantation genetic diagnosis or through amniocentesis. An image of disability is set at the birth of a newborn child. But predictions about any individual life are always hypothetical and often wrong. In interviewing hundreds of parents of children with disabilities, I found a recurring theme of indignation from parents whose children had achieved much more—or much less—than doctors had anticipated. A baby, disabled or not, is a cypher, and only time will show how and what he or she will do. Doctors who deliver prognostications are usually representing averages. On average, certain conditions bestow certain degrees of disability, but brains and bodies are highly adaptive, and the skills of an individual child can surprise everyone. It is a tough call for doctors. Creating an atmosphere of false hope can be catastrophic; it sets families up for renewed despair with every milestone their child misses. But presuming the worst often results in the worst results; low expectations can be a self-fulfilling prophecy. A tempered realism about the vagaries and uncertainties often obtains the best result, but parents crave assurances and doctors too often indulge that inclination.

The mother of a man with diastrophic dwarfism, a very disabling condition, described to me how for the first year of her son's life, every doctor she saw rattled off a catalogue of what was likely to go wrong and asked her if she was prepared to deal with it all. When her son was a year old, a doctor who specialized in skeletal dysplasias lifted the baby up, held him aloft in the light, and said, "Let me tell you. That's going to be a handsome young man one day." The rewarding life she was to have with her son began that very day, a fact she reflected on when we chatted at his joyous wedding years later. The expectations with which a child is raised may have a strongly determining effect on what that child can do. Parents must hope for the best but also believe that life will have meaning even with a child who achieves limited functioning. The process of forging meaning does wonders for both parents and child. A recent study looked at children with various complications at birth and found, simply, "The children of mothers who had tried harder to find meaning had a better developmental outcome." How we frame disability determines how we live it, and if it is defined as calamitous from the start, the job of finding meaning is steeper than it need be. The fact that you wouldn't have chosen something doesn't mean that you can't find joyful meaning in it.

Every condition manifests in a mix of inherent challenges,

access challenges, and social challenges. Many people with achondroplasia (the most common form of dwarfism) have spinal compression and need surgery for it. We can fix social attitudes toward people with dwarfism all we want, and spinal decompression procedures will neither be obviated nor become pleasant. They are an inherent challenge of the condition. Challenges of access are amply addressed by the Americans With Disabilities Act and we recognize the need for accommodations to address them, but though things are much better than they were on this front, problems persist. So someone with achondroplasia may be unable to reach the cereal at the local supermarket. The solution to this problem is not to make the LP (little person) taller, but to build grocery stores with lower shelving—or at least to give customers some tools or assistance that allow them to retrieve what they want to put in their cart. Because achondroplasia is a relatively infrequent disability, there are no standards for addressing high grocery shelves. That is a challenge of access.

The social challenges are the most pernicious. It is tough for dwarfs that people stare at them and try to make iPhone videos of them when they are quietly leading their regular lives. People try to joke with them; they say derogatory things in plain earshot. They plan parties at which dwarfs are the extraordinary entertainment. There is no escape from the intrusive exoticizing. These social problems of intractable rudeness are obdurate. An intellectually disabled person may not be able to parse difficult texts at the library; a physically disabled person may not be able to get up the front steps to that same library; someone with a speech impediment may be dealt with patronizingly there. We can't make good policy unless we acknowledge that all three challenges—inherent, access and social—are almost always in play.

Negative views of disability are deeply rooted in tradition. The evil of Shakespeare's Richard III was inseparable from his hunchback. The disabled body was morally suspect. In "Henry VI, Part 3," Gloucester (who would become Richard III) says bitterly, "Since the heavens have shaped my body so, / Let hell make crooked my mind to answer it." Disability was an invitation to degenerate behavior. He goes on, "And this word 'love,' which graybeards call divine, / Be resident in men like one another / And not in me: I am myself alone." To be found grotesque is often to become grotesque; we fit other people's perceptions of us and grow into what they see. Forced into isolation by a deformity, the disabled man is infected with rancor that has no other occasion. Though we've disavowed Shakespeare's association between deformity and evil, the burden of being perceived as different persists, and it can generate isolation and rage. The best solution to this problem is community, and this book is both the locus and the proof of community. That The New York Times published these stories points to the new ways communities are being built and acknowledged; and those who read them may find redemptive community in these words. This is not to say that if Richard III had belonged to a chat group of other hunchbacks he would have been a cheerful fellow, but only to comment that unmitigated outsiderness has always been poisonous and remains so.

The essays in this book do a double trick: They normalize disability and they exceptionalize it. Disabled lives are as valid as nondisabled lives, but they are not the same. This quest to assert equality without making false claims of equivalence finds itself in this series and its politics, and echoes the quest of the women's movement, the civil rights movement, and the gay rights movement to assert their legitimacy without melting into a bland sameness with the rest of the population. The idea that disability is an identity still comes as news to much of the general population and to many disabled people as well, but it has achieved an acceptance in the last decade or so that once seemed unimaginable. The disability Op-Ed series in The New York Times has been by disabled people and for both disabled people and a wider audience. Much of it is an act of translation between the experience of disabled people and the experience of nondisabled ones. Ability is both a selective and a temporary state; any individual can do only some of what other human beings can do, and over a lifetime, the level of ability generally starts low, builds to a prime, and then declines. Disabled people constitute the largest minority in America, but the disabled fail to speak with a single voice. Old men in wheelchairs too often deny their commonalities with children with autism or middle-aged people with Down syndrome.

Isolationism is a national policy of separating your country from dependence on others, and I believe it has been overplayed of late. It has its human equivalent in the elevation of personal independence: independence of children from parents, of parents from extended family, of extended family from the society around them. We admire the ability of people to stand on their own two feet and to function without reliance on social supports. Pundits disparage those who depend on public funding. But where has this modern, Western value originated?

Independence is not so brave a value as we often insist, and it is also almost impossible; we live in a collective fabric, all our lives entwined with the lives of others. Human beings are social animals. Disabled people are often dependent on other people, and in our lionization of self-sufficiency, we see that as a weakness. But to be more than usually dependent, or to be dependent on others for more of what one does is not to be reduced in value; dependency has its own particular poetry. It is a fundamental aspect of intimacy, a defining quality of love.

When I first came across inclusion and mainstreaming as educational strategies, I thought they must be lovely for the disabled people whose position was advanced. Separate education is never equal, and now people with disabilities would have access to high-quality teaching among the kind of people they'd be dealing with for the rest of their lives. But I thought it might be tough on the nondisabled people, whose progress would inevitably be slowed down by the accommodations that their disabled classmates required. Now, having been in many such classrooms, I can say that the primary advantage redounds to the nondisabled children, who grow up less afraid of difference than they would otherwise be, more receptive to the intense humanity of their fellow students. They do not think that independence is success and dependence is failure. This can allow them to be more willing to acknowledge their own dependence, to tolerate their own vulnerability.

Until Jason Kingsley, who has Down syndrome, began appearing on "Sesame Street" in the 1970s, there had been almost no disabled children publicly visible since the Victorian era, when the disabled were often sentimentalized and gathered at the family hearth. In the twentieth century, people whose children were disabled tended to hide them, seldom taking them into the market squares or shopping malls or restaurants or theaters where human beings come into contact with strangers. They were squirreled away at home or ferried to institutions, an exhausting embarrassment. Now, disabled people are more visible than ever. We live in a time of great social progress, when that visibility has been achieved—but we also live in a time of great medical progress, and at the same time that many forms of disability are being acknowledged as identities, they are becoming subject to cure. I believe in social progress and I believe in medical progress, but it would be tremendous for them to be more awake to each other. Disability may coexist with shocking ability; indeed, the shocking ability may rise in part from the depth of consciousness required of people who are disabled and who have to figure out an often bewildering world through their particular consciousness. To imagine, and I use the most obvious example, Stephen Hawking without disability is to imagine someone else entirely.

I come to this movement for rights through my struggle with depression, a mental illness that can earn you disability stripes. Depression's up side is substantial; I've learned a lot from my depression. If I had my life to do over, however, I'd wish it away. I pray that it never afflicts my children. I also belong, as we all do, to myriad other minorities. If I imagine myself without dyslexia, without ADD, without depression, without gayness, without near-sightedness, without orthostatic hypotension, without Jewishness, without white privilege, without prosopagnosia, then there's very little of me left. We are mostly an accumulation of strengths and weaknesses, of pathologized and nonpathologized conditions and identities. My grandmother used to say, "Everybody's got some-thing." So this book, though it is about disability, is really in many ways about how we seek for meaning in who we are rather than in who we might have wished to be. It may be easier in the United States as it's currently constructed to be white than it is to be of color, but most people of color do not spend their time wishing they had pale skin and golden hair. Women may know that men have more privilege, but women don't in general experience that differ-ence as one they would address by switching gender. We are our authentic selves, striving for justice, and the rest is commentary.

This book is written by people with disabilities, and is there-fore not representative of those disabled people who do not use language. Many who do not use spoken or written language com-municate through behavior or facial expression. But those who are in common parlance referred to as the "most disabled" are nearly voiceless, and we cannot guess what their inner life is like. Disabled people with access to language try to project those lives, but there is much that remains unknowable, even unimaginable. This book of words cannot speak for them. But it speaks with many voices of an astonishingly broad range of challenges and victories.

There's a lot of indignation in this collection, as disabled people are repeatedly denied accommodation and respect. There's a lot of sadness, too, often coincident with anger, as people find themselves marginalized and subject to prejudice. But overwhelming those hard emotions is self-belief, the conviction that disabled lives can be triumphant, and that such triumph is often sweetened by the difficulty of achieving it.

—Andrew Solomon

PREFACE

This book, "About Us," collects roughly 60 essays first published in The New York Times opinion series Disability. The series, which debuted in August 2016, was the first of its kind: a platform in a major news publication devoted to writing by and about people living with disabilities. In weekly essays over the two-year span this collection covers, the authors of Disability reached thousands, sometimes hundreds of thousands, of The New York Times readers through their stories, often igniting frank and impassioned conversations around topics and perspectives rarely aired in the media. Through their open and generous participation, these writers helped undo stereotypes and misperceptions, created unexpected human connections and established a space in which people with disabilities can be seen and heard as they are, not as they are perceived by others.

The authors of "About Us" represent a wide range of voices and experience. They include those with physical, motor, sensory and cognitive differences. They are students, artists, scholars, poets, novelists, journalists, doctors, activists and accomplished literary figures like the essayist Edward Hoagland and the neurologist and author Oliver Sacks. (I sometimes like to imagine Dr. Sacks in the afterlife, observing this project approvingly.)

You have probably noticed that the book's title has a familiar ring. It is derived from "Nothing about us without us," the motto of inclusion and self-representation widely adopted by the disability rights movement. It also stands as our guiding editorial principle.

By ensuring that people with disabilities tell their own stories, we intend to avoid and counter the sort of biased, simplified, often demeaning portrayals of them that are produced by an American popular culture designed by and for the nondisabled.

There is something else that distinguishes "About Us" from most available literature on disability. The works here are neither academic treatises nor political advocacy. Each piece is a personal account, a relevant, clearly written and accessible narrative—part storytelling, part argument, part oral history—intended for both general readers and those who wish to gain a deeper understanding of the lives and circumstances of people living with disabilities. They explore not only aspects of social justice and human ethics, but also revelatory moments that speak to the full human experience—first romance, childhood shame and isolation, discrimination, professional ambition, identity, child-bearing, parenting, aging and more.

It is important to note that the "us" in "About Us" is no fringe population. By many estimates roughly one in five Americans— about 60 million people—are living with a disability. It is a group legally defined to extend far beyond people with inherited genetic or congenital conditions to include those affected by age, injury, mental or physical illness or other life circumstances. That means that any one person can at any time enter the ranks of the disabled, and most of us certainly will. In this sense "About Us" is not just about that one in five; it is truly about *all* of us.

As the founding editor of the Times series (and co-editor of this book), I am often asked about its origin. Why *disability?* Why, in a media landscape in which virtually any subject is fair game, did we choose this one? Many wondered if I had a disability that compelled me to develop the series (I do not), or if disability had directly touched my friends or family (it has). These factors, however, were only peripheral.

There are instead a few simple answers to the essential question of *why.* The first motivation was journalistic. As an editor at a major media organization over the past decade, I was familiar with the significant flourishing of journalistic and literary voices from historically marginalized groups—the gay rights and marriage movement, Black Lives Matter, the LGBTQ and women's rights movements—but found no equivalent presence in the disability rights movement. In a very basic editorial sense, it was an area that needed coverage.

The second motivation is probably best described as literary. While I am well aware that concise, sharply argued op-eds are the heartbeat of any news opinion section, I hoped to create a project that would have long-term value, independent of any news cycle. Somewhere in the back of my mind was the echo of Ezra Pound's much quoted definition of literature—news that stays news. Over time, I came to believe that Disability would work best by pursuing a deeper, more personal sort of expression that might build familiarity, even intimacy, between reader and writer, without the social interference—habits, barriers and biases—that normally prevent such connection in public life. I began to imagine a space (in the case of our series, a digital one)—where that sort of unobstructed communication and communion could take place.

From the start that meant choosing writers and essays largely based on the traditional elements of literature—voice, narrative strength, storytelling skill. I found no shortage of terrific writers among those identifying as disabled. In fact, one of the surprise outcomes of the series was the energizing effect it seemed to have on the community of fiction writers, essayists, poets, artists and scholars with disabilities.

As my work in the series exposed me to the insights and ideas of our various authors, my own thinking about disability deepened and changed. I began to see disability not as a category, but rather a spectrum on which we all occupy a place. I began to understand disability itself as a "two-way street"—defined not just by a person's physical or biological makeup, but also by the degree to which social and structural barriers like lack of accessibility and accommodations prevent that person's full participation in society. Among readers, reactions like this have been common. I have heard directly from many readers about the profound intellectual, emotional and even spiritual effects that the series had on them.

It is an undeniable fact that most people are socially trained to look away from disability, to avoid any person who seems too "different" in appearance, speech, mannerism, body shape or size or behavior. The excuses are familiar: Direct contact with people who don't fit our ideas of sameness can be "awkward" or make us feel "overwhelmed." In social situations, "we don't know what to do," so we avoid them. By looking away—"not staring"—we are being "polite."

What the writers of "About Us" have accomplished in the course of this series, and in this book, is a subversion of these habitual avoidances. In telling their stories free of physical barriers, social habits, prejudices and customs, the authors have entered into direct, often intimate conversation with their readers, and the wider public.

I see—and you may, too—"About Us" as a collective act of social imagination. It makes a strong case for the dignity of all humans, but not by lecturing. It is a small but powerful contribution to the cause of greater understanding and community. It opens a door to the sort of full engagement with others that thinkers like the Jewish mystic and philosopher Martin Buber described as necessary to meaningful participation in society.

The work here is not merely testimony to the social, institutional and legal barriers that its authors have faced, but also to the resourcefulness, persistence and wit involved in thinking and acting their way past those barriers, and the eventual removal of them for all of us.

—Peter Catapano

INTRODUCTION

Living Well in a World Not Made for Us

"About Us: Essays from the Disability Series of The New York Times" brings us new stories about disability in today's world. And what's newest here is that people with disabilities are telling our own stories, both in the pages of The New York Times, and in this book. The series' authors delivered reports from the field, testimonies, protests and revelations about living with disabilities to millions of Times readers. In doing so, they helped reshape the national consciousness and conversation about the shared human condition we think of as disability.

This book *about us* and *by us* harkens to the unifying call of our civil rights movement—"Nothing About Us Without Us." Our stories are claims to self-representation and recognition that this slogan demands. "About Us" offers you an intimacy that comes through story. Our stories acknowledge how our distinctive perspectives as people with disabilities set the contours of our worldviews, actions and relations with one another.

Claiming an identity can be an act of self-knowledge and of generosity toward our interlocutors, letting them know how we understand ourselves and who we think we are. By telling our own stories, we rewrite the old scripts of disability that so many of us have had to live by because we haven't had any others. These stories are often surprising, even revelatory. We show the ways that living with disabilities shapes lives, that tired stereotypes are too simple, and that the struggles and pleasures of life with disabilities are both the same as and different from everyone else's. Our stories don't ask for sympathy, plead for inclusion or extol tolerance—as does so much traditional disability advocacy or advice from therapeutic, clinical or spiritual experts. We are the expert users of our own lives and makers of our own stories, self-advocates defining ourselves in all our distinctiveness and complexity.

Many of our lives run counter to the usual stories about disability as only bad news, the curse everyone wants to avoid. We do not necessarily understand our ways of being in the world as disadvantage, diminishment or distress. Such a worldview can be difficult to grasp for people who understand themselves as nondisabled because ours is a minority experience that the majority often find hard to imagine. Our stories here reach out to nondisabled readers, but they also let us look toward one another. These stories about us and by us help everyone better understand what emerges from navigating a world not made for us.

Perhaps the most significant contribution "About Us" offers is to humanize what could be the most human of experiences. Our conditions—whether intense or mundane, fleeting or enduring—are embedded in full lives that are as messy and measured as anyone's and that give meaning to our disabilities. We tell you what our lives are like, how they make sense to us, how we do things, and what's done to us. Ours are stories of human development, in which we may start out one way—seeing, hearing, walking, moving—and then shift suddenly or gradually into another mode of being that requires us to use the world differently. The long tradition from which everyone comes effaces the prevalence and inevitability of the human development that is disability, one we all transition into somehow, sometime. As one New York Times reader of the disability series commented, "There are two kinds of people in the world: the disabled and the not-yet-disabled."

Disability is a life task all people learn to navigate, one way or another. Few of us assume that we will need to adjust so fully to the barriers of getting through our days and carrying out what life expects from us. The not-yet-disabled must abide and accompany loved ones and family members who have entered into disability as they wait to join those of us who are already there. When we come to recognize that disability is with us, we will all need to know what's found in this book. Our stories here of disability lived deliberately, even if unwillingly, escort all of us in that shared human task.

The collective story The New York Times series on disability tells is not only how we live with the profusion of disabilities in our bodies and minds but also how we live with the social label "disabled." Because the arrival of disability is often random and precipitous, we are rarely prepared for the status change "disabled" forces upon us. The onset of disability can bring an abrupt dissonance between who we were yesterday and who we are today. An oncoming car in the wrong lane can transform the person we think we are today to a different one tomorrow. No other social identity category is so porous and unstable. In fact, most of us will live on both sides of the volatile line between disabled and non-disabled. Moving from the prestigious category of the normal and healthy into the social spaces where we have learned to think the abnormal and the ill reside is always unsettling, or worse, to one's sense of personal dignity.

No one easily embraces identifying or being identified with this deeply discredited and stigmatized group. Disability forces us to use not only our bodies or minds, but also the world itself, differently from how we may have used it before and from the way the nondisabled majority has built it. Many of our stories bear witness to this awkward shift away from what was quite recently a familiar and comfortable fit with both the material and social world. From the transition that disability occasions often comes the resourcefulness that has made many of us into agents for change, advocates for the political and social promises of the disability rights movement.

Indeed, the struggle to flourish in the category "disabled" is as much a part of the stories here as is the struggle to flourish with the bodies and minds we have. Disability often presents a tough situation semantically as well as materially. Many of the writers here wrestle with the very words of "disability," with whether we count ourselves or our particular embodiment as part of what the world considers "disabled" to mean and encompass. Some of us don't actually think of ourselves as disabled. We wonder whether stuttering, depression, anxiety, chronic pain or disfigurement are legitimate disabilities, alternately claiming and denying the category. Some of us don't consider ourselves disabled enough to receive the benefits or protections of the new disability laws. Others take exception to the low expectations implicit in legal protections. For all of us, the assumption that ours is a deficit mode of existence is an insult. Even though the anonymity of the unremarkable or the ordinary is a safe refuge, some of us disavow the prerogatives of normal. One "About Us" contributor, Ben Mattlin, strives instead to "like the disability that has contributed to who I am." Another, Jonathan Mooney, redefines "disability" with subtlety by telling readers: "I've come to believe that I did not have a disability, as it is common to say, but *experienced* disability in environments that could not accommodate and embrace my differences."

Those of us who wear the label "disabled" carry a heavy history. Even though human and civil rights–based precedent decree that we are both morally and legally of equal worth to our fellow citizens, assured of our rights, and protected under the law, a glance at the distant or even the recent history of people with disabilities reminds us of our grim vulnerability. The pronouncements of degeneracy, defect, unfitness and burden that confined us to asylums, hospitals, segregated schools and hidden back rooms are only a few decades in the past. In 1927, Supreme Court Justice Oliver Wendell Holmes authorized involuntary sterilization for people deemed "feebleminded," justifying that opinion by declaring that "Three generations of imbeciles are enough." People with Down syndrome, the first disability targeted for genetic detection and selective elimination in the 1960s, were at the time called "Mongoloid idiots," a diagnostic category fusing racial and disability discrimination to warrant permanent institutionalization. When Ed Roberts, the wheelchair-using disability rights activist and a founder of the independent living movement, enrolled at the University of California, Berkeley, in 1963, a headline in the Berkeley Gazette proclaimed, "Helpless cripple attends classes at UC."

The worldwide eugenics movement of the late nineteenth and early twentieth century turned medical science toward the enterprise of improving the human race by increasing the population of supposedly high-quality people and reducing the population of people those high-quality people deemed low-quality people. In the mid-twentieth century, extermination soon enough became the most efficient alternative to institutionalization of people that Nazi propaganda called "useless eaters." As Kenny Fries reminds us in his essay here, disabled people were the first targets for organized state-sponsored sterilization and euthanasia programs. The medical-scientific aim to make us "better" clumsily balances the conflict between the charge of medicine to "do good" and the caution to "do no harm."

Whereas cultural institutions such as medicine, war and industrialization make nondisabled people into disabled people all the time, they also develop technology, treatment and policies that attenuate the disjuncture between our bodies and minds and a world built for the normal. The eugenic aspirations of our current moment use nothing as crude as gas chambers to improve the human race, but nonetheless assiduously advance medical normalization and experimentation, prenatal testing and selective termination, genetic modification, physician-aided dying, withholding treatment and resource distribution to eradicate disability—and, often enough, people with disabilities. A widely shared philosophy from practical ethicists such as Peter Singer provocatively supports a liberal eugenics that permits euthanizing certain disabled newborns. Many of the writers collected here live uneasily with medical conditions explicitly targeted for extermination in the past and for elimination today.

Most of us have lived on both sides of the cultural and political transformation of the disability rights movement that changed our understanding of our bodies and minds from medical conditions to political affiliation. This shift from being medical to political subjects recognized us as "people with disabilities," a political designation created through a series of policies, laws and covenants ranging from human rights declarations to equal education policy, architectural barriers removal acts, the Americans With Disabilities Act of 1990 and 2009, to the United Nations Convention on the Rights of People with Disabilities—all aimed toward disability justice. Many of our stories acknowledge the residue of the old exclusions that kept us out of schools, workplaces, public transportation and civic life in general and recognize, even celebrate, our new opportunities and the paths—quite literally—that we now understand ourselves as having the right to access. We lament the barriers that still block inclusion, and we hail the possibilities available to us.

As a distinctly modern identity, "disability" is a group affiliation endowed with political rights that we can claim and that can claim us. Many of us have invested in this identity as persons with disabilities and detail the benefits, even pleasures, of living with disabilities as people with disabilities. We don't spend time wishing to be someone else but instead put our energies into flourishing as we are. Some of us relish the challenges of such a life; others are demoralized. For some of us disability is neutral variation; for others, it is cultural membership; for still others, it is pathology. Some of us resist the calls to such an affiliation, chafing against the stereotypes of inspiration, sympathy, or a toxic political correctness that flattens out individuality.

All of us have thrived, however we could, and our stories tell how we have managed, not in spite of our disabilities, but often because of our disabilities. We have not so much overcome as worked with bodies, minds and sensibilities that often put us at odds with our world. Not all of us are satisfied with our lives; indeed, our stories span exasperation to outrage, grief to desolation, and bafflement to chaos about the ways we get through life.

The writers here certainly do not represent the wide range of Americans with disabilities. What links us together is that all of us have had access to educational opportunities that in the past, and even now, have been withheld from people with disabilities. The right to an equal and appropriate education that became available to people with disabilities starting in the 1970s has extended to us the possibility to accrue cultural and economic capital from which we've made good lives and gathered the resources to navigate the inevitable limitations and troubles of the human condition. Education and the goods it brings to anyone provides us an eloquence widely shared by human beings both disabled and nondisabled through which we express distinctive ways we live with disabilities. We are writers, all.

Many of our readers found an unexpected kinship with us. Our stories recognized their transitions into disability in their own lives and affirmed how they have been touched by, often shaken by, disability in some way. "I realized that I'm not alone in being alone," one reader commented. Many readers thanked us for bringing forward topics and perspectives completely fresh to them. Someone wrote to me with gratitude for giving them an entirely new way of looking at disability. The singularity of our experiences spoke to many readers. One said that my story captured their own experience in a way they'd never seen before. Another wrote to me that my "insights brought . . . tears of recognition and sympathy" because he had never met another person with a disability like his own. Many comments were cheers of solidarity, from, "You go, girl!" to "Beautiful writing. Please, more." Some readers offered the wisdom of long proficiency: "Life, once formed, is tenacious" and "Normal is being alive, not the shape of our bodies." One man wrote to me, "I keep telling people they do not understand what it is like to actually BE disabled until you ARE."

Other readers, however, disagreed with our claims or resisted our offered alignments. "No, You are not disabled," one commenter pronounced to a writer questioning the boundaries of disability categories. Some dissent was stronger: "There is NOTHING good about becoming disabled. N O T O N E T H I N G!" Another avowed, "You.do.not.know.the.whole.story." One reader deemed disability "too absurd a form of delusional identity politics." Taken together, the comments on The New York Times website for the series form a communal call and response to becoming disabled, living with disabilities and knowing the ways of being we think of as disabled.

"About Us" arranges the more than sixty essays here in categories that focus on enduring themes and tasks of living that give meaning and purpose to the lives of all people—beginning with "Justice" and ending with "Joy."

"Justice" gathers stories that reflect how many of us have come to understand being disabled as a social, even political, situation more than a medical condition. The first-person stories here collectively trace a history of disability discrimination and liberation in the twentieth century, from the eugenic extermination in the Holocaust to the struggle for political equality and the paths toward its realization at the end of the twentieth century and into the next. Stories of the successes and failures of accessibility, protections, autonomy and entitlements interweave here. We see protests against the way popular culture mocks mental illness, the challenges wheelchair users face, our need for adequate healthcare provision and how the protections of the Americans With Disabilities Act can be a lifesaving measure for people with minimal consciousness. Such an emerging concept of disability justice has shaped all of the lives of the writers in "About Us."

"Belonging" considers who we are and how "disabled" draws us together, gladly or hesitantly, into a community. These stories range across the experiences of people who live with deafness or blindness, who use crutches, tic or twitch, have genetic conditions or unusual appearances. Taken together, our embrace or resistance reveals not just the variation of human ways of being that make up disability categories, but they also tell more deeply a range of our own responses to being considered "disabled," how we understand ourselves as people with disabilities and the tribes with which we make affiliation.

"Working" shows how we make things and how we do our jobs. Before the disability rights movement, attitudes and inaccessible built environments excluded us from the benefits and responsibilities of meaningful work, for the most part. Now that many of us have gained access to education and employment opportunities, we have reshaped the workplace, the workforce and the marketplace, locally and globally. Our experiences of living with disabilities structure how we work—from doctoring to lawyering—and what we make in our work as artists, writers, or teachers. We are expert users, lifehackers, of situations into which we fit uneasily, transforming the work world with our presence and distinctive expertise.

"Navigating" details how we use tools, strategies, and innovations to get through our days. Our technology has moved from medical equipment to access technologies. The wheelchairs to which so many of us were previously "confined" or "bound" have become now at once the symbol and reality of our entrance into public spaces and public life. Ours are stories of ingenuity born of opportunity and restriction as we follow along and lead the way out and about in the world with our white canes, walking aids, ramps, high-tech limbs, implants.

"Coping" reveals some of our struggles and the ways we survive them. Living in a world not built for us can be an occasion for resourcefulness and a source of frustration. These stories show that living with a disability can be hard work; health maintenance can be complicated; the burden of stigma can be heavy; managing psychoemotional changes can be wearing; traversing the breach between us and the nondisabled can attenuate our energy and resources. We show you how we endure and maintain our dignity in the face of these tasks.

"Love" offers tender, heartening, exasperating, and ordinary love stories and what's particular about how we live them. Because the way all of us live now tends toward the inherent isolation individualism brings, finding and sustaining the human connections of love challenge all modern people. Modern mating rituals such as online dating and our overvaluing of standardized appearance and upscaled conformity can be barriers to making lasting love in all its varieties for people with disabilities. These stories show us some of the forms of modern love people with disabilities cultivate.

"Family" attends to how disability shapes our made and chosen families and the intergenerational dynamics disability introduces. Disability connects families in distinctive ways. These stories present the complexities of how genetic conditions bond parent and child; how we navigate corrosive connections such as blame, guilt, and recrimination within families; what comforts we find in similarities and differences forged by inherited or congenital disabilities; and what we give to and take from one another in the exchanges of care and dependence that come with the bodies and minds we inhabit.

"Joy" illuminates how we relish and revel in our lives as people with disabilities. Perhaps the most unjustified stereotype about disability is that our lives are filled with relentless and unaccountable suffering. While all the stories collected here counter that assumption, the ones we leave you with bring forward the distinctive joys that can come to lives lived well with disabilities. Deafness, we learn here, is not the absence of sound but rather an opportunity for creative meaning making or a fresh way to know music. Blindness can be an opportunity for imagination that the ease of sightedness blunts. Chronic illness presents satisfying, if less traveled, paths we would not otherwise have taken. Often harrowing experiences of neurodiversity or other psychosocial disturbances connect us to historical figures with whom we may have little else in common. No life is without sadness, suffering or struggle. And like everyone else, we've all had our allotment. The stories we offer you as our closing amply witness the often unexpected entanglement of joy with difficulty, pleasure with distress, accommodation with resistance. They show you how all of us writers here cultivate joy where and how we are able.

This book is a gift to us all. Our stories testify to our persistence, to getting through our lives with dignity and generosity toward our fellow humans, disabled and nondisabled alike. As Laurie Clements Lambeth clarifies here, "All creatures who persist are whole." We are whole not through our bodies and minds but through our continuing urge to be, to live fully as we are and who we are in a world that does not expect us and is often not made for us. Our collected stories here are not a lament or reproach, but an invitation to readers to rebuild along with us the world we share and live in together. There is much work to do to realize together the promises of the disability rights movement and what it makes in our communities and larger world. "About Us" witnesses the rich particularity of the lives we have made in this moment in this place, and it intimates what can come from our continued persistence.

—Rosemarie Garland-Thomson

I

JUSTICE

Becoming Disabled

ROSEMARIE GARLAND-THOMSON

NOT LONG AGO, A GOOD FRIEND OF MINE SAID SOMETHING REVEALING to me: "I don't think of you as disabled," she confessed.

I knew exactly what she meant; I didn't think of myself as disabled until a few decades ago, either, even though my two arms have been pretty significantly asymmetrical and different from most everybody else's my whole life.

My friend's comment was meant as a compliment, but followed a familiar logic—one that African-Americans have noted when their well-meaning white friends have tried to erase the complications of racial identity by saying, "I don't think of you as black," or when a man compliments a woman by saying that he thinks of her as "just one of the guys."

This impulse to rescue people with disabilities from a discredited identity, while usually well meaning, is decidedly at odds with the various pride movements we've come to know in recent decades. Slogans like "Black Is Beautiful" and "We're Here, We're Queer, Get Used to It!" became transformative taunts for generations of people schooled in the self-loathing of racism, sexism and heterosexism. Pride movements were the psychoemotional equivalents of the anti-discrimination and desegregation laws that asserted the rights of full citizenship to women, gay people, racial minorities and other groups. More recently, the Black Lives Matter and the LGBTQ rights movement have also taken hold.

Yet pride movements for people with disabilities—like Crip Power or Mad Pride—have not gained the same sort of traction in the American consciousness. Why? One answer is that we have a much clearer collective notion of what it means to be a woman or an African-American, gay or transgender person than we do of what it means to be disabled.

A person without a disability may recognize someone using a wheelchair, a guide dog or a prosthetic limb, or someone with Down syndrome, but most don't conceptualize these people as having a shared social identity and a political status. "They" merely seem to be people to whom something unfortunate has happened, for whom something has gone terribly wrong. The one thing most people do know about being disabled is that they don't want to be that.

Yet disability is everywhere once you start noticing it. A simple awareness of who we are sharing our public spaces with can be revelatory. Wheelchair users or people with walkers, hearing aids, canes, service animals, prosthetic limbs or breathing devices may seem to appear out of nowhere, when they were in fact there all the time.

A mother of a 2-year-old boy with dwarfism who had begun attending Little People of America events summed this up when she said to me with stunned wonder, "There are a lot of them!" Until this beloved child unexpectedly entered her family, she had no idea that achondroplasia is the most common form of short stature or that most people with the condition have average-size parents. More important, she probably did not know how to request the accommodations, access the services, enter the communities or use the laws that he needs to make his way through life. But because he is hers and she loves him, she will learn a lot about disability.

The fact is, most of us will move in and out of disability in our lifetimes, whether we do so through illness, an injury or merely the process of aging.

The World Health Organization defines disability as an umbrella term that encompasses impairments, activity limitations and participation restrictions that reflect the complex interaction between "features of a person's body and features of the society in which he or she lives." The Americans With Disabilities Act tells us that disability is "a physical or mental impairment that substantially limits one or more major life activities."

Obviously, this category is broad and constantly shifting, so exact statistics are hard to come by, but the data from our most reliable sources is surprising. The Centers for Disease Control and Prevention estimates that one in five adults in the United States is living with a disability. The National Organization on Disability says there are 56 million disabled people (many estimates are higher). Indeed, people with disabilities are the largest minority group in the United States, and as new disability categories such as neurodiversity, psychiatric disabilities, disabilities of aging and learning disabilities emerge and grow, so does that percentage.

Disability growth areas—if you will—include diagnostic categories such as depression, anxiety disorders, anorexia, cancers, traumatic brain injuries, attention-deficit disorder, autoimmune disease, spinal cord injuries, autistic spectrum disabilities and dementia. Meanwhile, whole categories of disability and populations of people with certain disabilities have vanished or diminished significantly in the 20th century with improved public health measures, disease prevention and increased public safety.

Because almost all of us will experience disability sometime in our lives, having to navigate one early in life can be a great advantage. Because I was born with six fingers altogether and one quite short arm, I learned to get through the world with the body I had from the beginning. Such a misfit between body and world can be an occasion for resourcefulness. Although I certainly recognized that the world was built for what I call the fully fingered, not for my body, I never experienced a sense of losing capacity, and adapted quite readily, engaging with the world in my preferred way and developing practical workarounds for the life demands my body did not meet. (I used talk-to-text technology to write this essay, for example.)

Still, most Americans don't know how to be disabled. Few of

us can imagine living with a disability or using the technologies that disabled people often need. Since most of us are not born into disability but enter into it as we travel through life, we don't get acculturated the way most of us do in our race or gender. Yet disability, like any challenge or limitation, is fundamental to being human—a part of every life. Clearly, the border between "us" and "them" is fragile. We just might be better off preparing for disability than fleeing from it.

Yet even talking about disability can be a fraught experience. The vocabulary of this status is highly charged, and for even the most well-meaning person, a conversation can feel like stepping into a maze of courtesy, correctness and possible offense. When I lecture about disability, someone always wants to know—either defensively, earnestly or cluelessly—the "correct" way to refer to this new politicized identity.

What we call ourselves can also be controversial. Different constituencies have vibrant debates about the politics of self-naming. "People first" language asserts that if we call ourselves "people with disabilities," we put our humanity first and consider our impairment a modification. Others claim disability pride by getting our identity right up front, making us "disabled people." Others, like many sign language users, reject the term "disability."

The old way of talking about disability as a curse, tragedy, misfortune or individual failing is no longer appropriate, but we are unsure about what more progressive, more polite, language to use. "Crippled," "handicapped" and "feebleminded" are outdated and derogatory. Many pre-Holocaust eugenic categories that were indicators for state-sponsored sterilization or extermination policies— "idiot," "moron," "imbecile" and even "mentally retarded"—have been discarded in favor of terms such as "developmentally delayed" or "intellectually disabled." In 2010, President Obama signed Rosa's Law, which replaced references to "mental retardation" with "intellectual disability" in federal statutes.

The author and scholar Simi Linton writes about learning to be disabled in a hospital after a spinal cord injury—not by way of her rehabilitation but rather by bonding with other young people new to disability. She calls this entering into community "claiming disability." In "Sight Unseen," an elegant explication of blindness and sight as cultural metaphors, Georgina Kleege wryly suggests the difference between medical low vision and blindness as a cultural identity by observing that "Writing this book made me blind," a process she calls gaining blindness rather than losing sight.

Like them, I had no idea until the 1980s what it meant to be disabled, that there was a history, culture and politics of disability. Without a disability consciousness, I was in the closet.

Since that time, other people with disabilities have entered the worlds in which I live and work, and I have found community and developed a sturdy disability identity. I have changed the way I see and treat myself and others. I have taken up the job of teaching disability studies and bioethics as part of my work. I have learned to be disabled.

What has been transformed is not my body, but my consciousness.

As we manage our bodies in environments not built for them, the social barriers can sometimes be more awkward than the physical ones. Confused responses to racial or gender categories can provoke the question "What are you?" Whereas disability interrogations are "What's wrong with you?" Before I learned about disability rights and disability pride, which I came to by way of the women's movement, I always squirmed out a shame-filled, "I was born this way." Now I'm likely to begin one of these uncomfortable encounters with "I have a disability," and to complete it with "and these are the accommodations I need." This is a claim to inclusion and right to access resources.

This coming out has made possible what a young graduate student with a disability said to me after I gave a lecture at her university. She said that she understood now that she had a right to be in the world.

We owe much of this progress to the Americans With Disabilities

Act of 1990 and the laws that led up to it. Starting in the 1960s, a broad disability rights movement encouraged legislation and policy that gradually desegregated the institutions and spaces that had kept disabled people out and barred them from exercising the privileges and obligations of full citizenship. Education, transportation, public spaces and work spaces steadily transformed so that people with disabilities came out of hospitals, asylums, private homes and special schools into an increasingly rebuilt and reorganized world.

That changed landscape is being reflected politically, too, so much so that when Donald Trump mocked the movement of a disabled reporter, most of the country reacted with shock and outrage at his blatant discrimination, and that by the time the Democratic National Convention rolled round, it seemed natural to find the rights and dignity of people with disabilities placed front and center. Hillary Clinton's efforts early in her career to secure the right to an education for all disabled children was celebrated; Tom Harkin, the former Iowa senator and an author of the Americans With Disabilities Act, marked the law's 26th anniversary and called for improvements to it. People with disabilities were featured speakers, including Anastasia Somoza, who received an ovation for her powerful speech. President Obama, in his address, referred to "black, white, Latino, Asian, Native American; young, old; gay, straight; men, women, folks with disabilities, all pledging allegiance, under the same proud flag."

Becoming disabled demands learning how to live effectively as a person with disabilities, not just living as a disabled person trying to become nondisabled. It also demands the awareness and cooperation of others who don't experience these challenges. Becoming disabled means moving from isolation to community, from ignorance to knowledge about who we are, from exclusion to access, and from shame to pride.

The Nazis' First Victims Were
the Disabled

KENNY FRIES

I SIT FACING THE YOUNG GERMAN NEUROLOGIST, ACROSS A SMALL TABLE IN a theater in Hamburg, Germany. I'm here giving one-on-one talks called "The Unenhanced: What Has Happened to Those Deemed 'Unfit'," about my research on Aktion T4, the Nazi "euthanasia" program to exterminate the disabled.

"I'm afraid of what you're going to tell me," the neurologist says.

I'm not surprised. I've heard similar things before. But this time is different—the young man sitting across from me is a doctor. Aktion T4 could not have happened without the willing participation of German doctors.

I have a personal stake in making sure this history is remembered. In 1960, I was born missing bones in both legs. At the time, some thought I should not be allowed to live. Thankfully, my parents were not among them.

I first discovered that people with disabilities were sterilized and killed by the Nazis when I was a teenager, watching the TV miniseries "Holocaust" in 1978. But it would be years before I understood the connections between the killing of the disabled and the killing of Jews and other "undesirables," all of whom were, in one way or another, deemed "unfit."

The neurologist does not know much about what I'm telling him. While he does know that approximately 300,000 disabled people were killed in T4 and its aftermath, he doesn't know about the direct connection between T4 and the Holocaust. He doesn't know that it was at Brandenburg, the first T4 site, where methods of mass killing were tested, that the first victims of Nazi mass killings were the disabled, and that its personnel went on to establish and run the extermination camps at Treblinka, Belzec and Sobibor.

Three years earlier, when I first arrived in Germany, I was consistently confronted with the treatment of those with disabilities under the Third Reich. But I soon realized I had to go back even further. In the 1920s, the disabled were mistreated, sterilized, experimented on and killed in some German psychiatric institutions. In 1920, the psychiatrist Alfred Hoche and the jurist Karl Binding published their treatise, "Permitting the Destruction of Unworthy Life," which became the blueprint for the exterminations of the disabled carried out by the Third Reich.

In Dr. Ewald Melzer's 1923 survey of the parents of the disabled children in his care, they were asked: "Would you agree definitely to a painless shortcut of your child's life, after it is determined by experts that it is incurably stupid?" The results, which surprised Dr. Melzer, were published in 1925: 73 percent responded they were willing to have their children killed if they weren't told about it.

I am also Jewish. At the Karl Bonhoeffer psychiatric hospital in the Berlin suburb of Wittenau, where the exhibition "A Double Stigma: The Fate of Jewish Psychiatric Patients" was held, I learned about, as the exhibition title suggests, how Jewish patients were doubly stigmatized by being separated from other patients, denied pastoral care, and were cared for not at the expense of the Reich but by Jewish organizations. Jewish patients were singled out for early extermination; by December 1942, the destruction of the Jewish patient population at Wittenau was complete.

The young neurologist in Hamburg did not know this history.

It is only at the end of my talk with the neurologist that I notice he wears a hearing aid. I want to ask if he knows about "100 Percent," the film produced by deaf Germans to show they could assimilate and be productive citizens who worked. Did he know the hereditary deaf were singled out not only by the German authorities but also by those with acquired deafness who tried to save themselves? Too often, even those of us with disabilities do not know our own history.

Not many people know about disability history in the United States. They do not know that in the United States in 1927, Justice Oliver Wendell Holmes wrote that "three generations of imbeciles are enough" as part of his opinion in Buck v. Bell, in which the Supreme Court ruled that compulsory sterilization of the "unfit" was constitutional. This decision has never been expressly overturned.

Many Americans still do not know about the so-called "ugly laws," which in many states, beginning in the late 1860s, deemed it illegal for persons who were "unsightly or unseemly" to appear in public. The last of these laws was not repealed until 1974.

Why is it important to know this history? We often say what happened in Nazi Germany couldn't happen here. But some of it, like the mistreatment and sterilization of the disabled, did happen here.

A reading of Hoche and Binding's "Permitting the Destruction of Unworthy Life" shows the similarity between what they said and what exponents of practical ethics, such as Peter Singer, say about the disabled today. As recently as 2015, Singer, talking with the radio host Aaron Klein on his show, said, "I don't want my health insurance premiums to be higher so that infants who can experience zero quality of life can have expensive treatments."

These philosophers talk about the drain on "resources" caused by lives lived with a disability, which eerily echoes what Hoche and Binding wrote about the "financial and moral burden" on "a person's family, hospital, and state" caused by what they deem lives "unworthy of living."

Experts point out the recent Republican health care proposals would strip Medicaid funding that helps the elderly, the poor and the disabled live healthier and more dignified lives. A recent New York Times article quoted the Rev. Susan Flanders, a retired

Episcopal priest, as saying: "What we're paying for is something that many people wouldn't want if they had a choice. It's hundreds of dollars each day that could go towards their grandchildren's education or care for the people who could get well."

In the article, Flanders, whose father had Alzheimer's, is described as "utterly unafraid to mix money into the conversation about the meaning of life when the mind deteriorates." Practical ethicists are similarly unafraid to do this. As were the Nazis. Third Reich school textbooks included arithmetic problems on how much it would cost to care for a person with a disability for a lifetime.

Three years ago, I was the only visitor at a museum dedicated to the history of the Reinickendorf area of Berlin. The museum building was once part of Wiesengrund, which, in 1941, housed the "wards for expert care" of the Municipal Hospital for Children.

Down a hall with fluorescent lighting, in a white-walled room, were 30 wooden cribs. On each of the cribs was a history of a child, some as young as a few months old. This was the room in which these infants and children were experimented on and killed: the 30-bed Ward 3, the "ward for expert care" at Wiesengrund.

My heart raced; my breath shortened. I couldn't stay in that room for long. The room evoked the first four weeks of my own life spent in an incubator. Nobody knew if I would live or die.

What kind of society do we want to be? Those of us who live with disabilities are at the forefront of the larger discussion of what constitutes a valued life. What is a life worth living? Too often, the lives of those of us who live with disabilities are not valued, and feared. At the root of this fear is misunderstanding, misrepresentation and a lack of knowledge of disability history and, thus, disabled lives.

Mental Illness Is Not a Horror Show

ANDREW SOLOMON

A NEW VIRTUAL-REALITY ATTRACTION PLANNED FOR KNOTT'S BERRY Farm in Buena Park, California, was announced in September 2016 in advance of the peak haunted-house season. The name, "Fear VR 5150," was significant. The number 5150 is the California psychiatric involuntary commitment code, used for a mentally ill person who is deemed a danger to himself or others.

Upon arrival in an ersatz "psychiatric hospital exam room," VR 5150 visitors would be strapped into a wheelchair and fitted with headphones. "The VR headset puts you in the middle of the action inside the hospital," an article in The Orange County Register explained. "One patient seems agitated and attempts to get up from a bed. Security officers try to subdue him. A nurse gives you a shot (which you will feel), knocking you out. When you wake up in the next scene, all hell has broken loose. Look left, right and down, bloody bodies lie on the floor. You hear people whimpering in pain." Knott's Berry Farm is operated by Ohio-based Cedar Fair Entertainment Company, and Fear VR 5150 was to be featured at two other Cedar Fair parks as well.

Almost simultaneously, two similar attractions were started at Six Flags. A news release for one explained: "Our new haunted house brings you face-to-face with the world's worst psychiatric patients. Traverse the haunted hallways of Dark Oaks Asylum and try not to bump into any of the grunting inmates around every turn. Maniacal inmates yell out from their bloodstained rooms and deranged guards wander the corridors in search of those who have escaped."

The Orange County branch of the National Alliance on Mental Illness sprang into action, and Doris Schwartz, a Westchester, N.Y.-based mental-health professional, immediately emailed a roster of 130 grass-roots activists, including me, many of whom flooded Cedar Fair and Six Flags with phone calls, petitions and emails. After some heated back-and-forth, Fear VR 5150 was shelved, and Six Flags changed the mental patients in its maze into zombies.

As both a psychiatric patient and a professor of clinical psychology, I was saddened to see painful lived experiences transmogrified into spooky entertainment. I was also unnerved to consider that I was someone else's idea of a ghoul, a figure more or less interchangeable with a zombie.

I became severely, clinically depressed for the first time in 1994. I was unable to speak, unable to get out of bed, unable to function in the world, and I thought of suicide constantly. I was afraid all the time but didn't know what I was afraid of; I was numb to my own emotions and stripped of vitality.

I have mostly done better these last two decades through the rigors of intensive treatment by both a psychoanalyst and a psychopharmacologist. I now take a cocktail of five medications and I go to therapy weekly. My mental illness is largely (though not entirely) under control, but as my therapist pointed out recently when I was cavalier about some warning signs, "In this room, Andrew, we never forget that you are entirely capable of taking the express elevator to the bargain basement of mental health."

I wrote about my experiences with depression in a book, "The Noonday Demon," and spoke about them in a TED talk, and I now get floods of mail from people who are dealing with mental illness—most of them isolated, terrified and bewildered; many of them unable to access the kind of decent care that has been so transformative for me.

For those of us with firsthand experience with mental illness—

especially those who have experienced trauma in a mental hospital—such entertainment ventures cut much too close to the bone. When my mother was dying of cancer, she was admitted to some miserable wards, but I find it hard to envision a Halloween event at which you would pretend to be getting chemotherapy and vomiting constantly while surrounded by patients driven into the quasi-dementia that comes of unremitting pain.

I have a pretty good sense of humor about myself. We all use the language of mental illness cavalierly. We say that our parents or our kids are driving us crazy; we complain we will soon go mad if the traffic doesn't clear; we accuse Donald Trump of having a personality disorder (which, whether accurate or not, is still intended as a disparagement). But I have also spent a lifetime trying to laugh when a friend has driven me past a psychiatric hospital and commented on the loons inside, to crack a smile when people have expressed their emotional extravagance with a jest about suicide.

Sanity and mental illness lie on a spectrum, and most people occasionally cross over from one side to the other. It's the proximity of mental illness rather than its obscurity that makes it so scary. But it should be scary in a "fix the broken care system" way or in a "figure out the brain's biology" way, and not in a "scream for laughs" kind of way.

The rhetoric with which Cedar Fair attempted to mollify the activists was troubling. The company wrote by way of explanation, "Our evening attractions are designed to be edgy, and are aimed at an adult-only audience." But "edgy" is not in general a euphemism for "stigmatizing of a disenfranchised population," and the defense that the attraction was for adults only seemed a very token mitigation—as though adults were not the progenitors of most chauvinism and hatred.

The attractions at Cedar Fair and Six Flags were not intended as representations of what mental illness is really like; they were incidentally demeaning, rather than willfully so. But how readily do such lapses approximate hate speech? And with what potential to provoke misunderstanding, fear and even harm to people with few defenses?

The misperception that mentally ill people are inherently dangerous is one of the most treacherous ideas in circulation about us. It surfaces widely every time a mass shooter is on the loose, and results in the subjugation of people who are not menacing in any way.

I recognize the free-speech claim that individuals and entertainment companies have every right to demean people with mental illnesses, but these representations have very real consequences— the stigmatization of the mentally ill, and the prejudice, poor treatment and violations of their rights that naturally follow.

Other people's fear of us can have terrible consequences. There are regular reports of police who respond aggressively or violently to the erratic behavior of mentally ill people, whether they are armed or not—the killing of Deborah Danner, a woman with schizophrenia, by a New York City police officer in October 2016 being just one recent example. There are more mentally ill people in our prison system than in our health care system.

It is possible to honor the power of burlesque even as we insist on respect for people who are too frequently harmed by it. In some hypothetical Venn diagram, there is an extravagant overlap between fun and cruelty. Slapstick, farce, satire—all these involve laughing at people who are slipping on a banana peel, or knocking their teeth in, or sitting down on a chair that isn't there to find themselves splayed on the floor. We laugh at big noses or flat noses, at vulgarity and buffoonery, at politics antithetical to our own. Clowns did this creepy work before there were creepy clowns on the loose.

I think of the effect these attractions would have not only on people without mental illnesses, who might be inspired to patronize, shun or even harm those of us who do have them, but also on the large portion of the American population who battle these challenges daily. Will they be more hesitant to come out about a psychiatric diagnosis? Will they be less likely to check themselves in for care? The injury is not only disrespect from the outside, but also a terrible doubting from within.

Our nation is in a moment when prejudice runs riot. Assertions of strength have often overtaken moral righteousness in the public imagination; success has been posited as incompatible with empathy. That rejection of empathy is an authentic poison, pressing some people to understand themselves as less human than others, a danger associated with a proliferation of suicides. It's hard to think well of yourself in a world that sees you as a threat.

Disability and the Right to Choose

JENNIFER BARTLETT

AS A YOUNG WOMAN, I HAD NO PARTICULAR DESIRE TO BE A MOTHER. I was neither for nor against having and raising a child, and as things were at the time, the opportunity had not presented itself. That changed when I was 29 and met Jim, the man who would become my husband. In 2002, not long after we married, I gave birth to my son.

In my 20s, I was neutral about parenthood partly because, as a woman with cerebral palsy, I was spared the usual intrusive questioning and expectations about having children that most women are subject to. People never pressured me to have children; they just assumed that I could not. In fact, it became clear very fast that women like me are expected *not* to reproduce. Now, in my 40s, I find these attitudes ignorant and prejudicial, but as a young woman, it seemed like a bit of freedom to be excused from the usual problems women complain about.

My disability is not genetic and it does not hamper pregnancy. Being pregnant was physically, emotionally and spiritually easy for me, but socially, it was complicated. Moving around in New York City as a pregnant woman with a disability opened me up for constant commentary. I am used to having my body be an object of attention. The real difficulty came from elsewhere—it was dealing with the medical establishment during my pregnancy that I was not prepared for.

Navigating the medical system as a pregnant woman is difficult;

as a disabled pregnant woman, it is nearly impossible. The first ob/gyn I went to told me condescendingly, "You sure know what's going on for someone in your condition." By "condition" she meant cerebral palsy.

She referred me to her colleague to get a sonogram because the clinic did not have the necessary equipment. This doctor was more respectful, so I wanted to be under his care. He told me that he could not treat me because it would be unethical "to take work" from his colleague.

I found a third doctor. This doctor was very traditional and although she did not infantilize me, there was a conflict because I wanted to have natural childbirth, and this was not in her vocabulary. In fact, she called my birth plan a "wish list." As my pregnancy developed, after taking a Bradley class and hiring a doula, I became more and more adamant about natural childbirth. At one point, I called the now-defunct Elizabeth Seton Natural Birth Center in Manhattan in an attempt to get a midwife. Without even an examination, I was told that the center would not take me as a client because I was "high risk." When I protested, the midwife told me if a woman at the center had trouble during labor, she would have to walk to the nearby hospital. There was no possibility that this was the case, but she managed to get rid of me. I had no choice but to stay with the third doctor.

In my fifth month of pregnancy, my doctor sent me to the hospital to have a transvaginal ultrasound to "check" the fetus. My doctor did not give the reason for the procedure or what it would determine. I later learned that in addition to determining the viability of the pregnancy, this type of ultrasound is used to detect Down syndrome and other birth "defects." I was already beginning to understand the ways in which modern medicine could be used to devalue, or even weed out, people with disabilities.

When I got pregnant, my husband and I discussed what we would do if our child had a disability. I didn't have any anxiety about it. In some ways, I viewed the possibility as an opportunity.

If my son ended up with cerebral palsy, he would be like me. If he ended up with a different disability, we would have a chance to see the world in a different light. Either way, there was no question in my mind that I would not have an abortion, no matter what the circumstance. We wanted our son, whether or not he had a disability. As it turned out, he did not.

In 2004, when my son was 3, I read an article in The New York Times that deeply upset me and has stayed with me. In it, Amy Harmon wrote about fetal genetic testing and the hundreds of "defects" that, even then, could be predicted before birth (this technology has since evolved rapidly, as we know). If an abnormality is detected, parents must make the decision whether to continue with the pregnancy or abort. One woman, with a genetic condition that caused her to have an extra finger, which she'd had surgically removed, chose to end two of her pregnancies because tests detected her fetuses' having the same condition. This instance is the extreme, but it is by no means an exception.

I support legal abortion and am not criticizing women who have made the difficult decision to terminate a pregnancy because of a disabled fetus. There are situations in which the life of the child would be so painful and short that abortion would be the most compassionate option.

I do believe, however, that aborting a fetus with a disability should not be a given. In his book "Far From the Tree," Andrew Solomon theorizes that families might abort fetuses if their sexual orientation could be determined. What he is touching upon is that there is sometimes a social and prejudicial component in the decision making. (We already know this danger is real; gender-selective abortions still take place in the hundreds of thousands in India and China each year, and in lesser numbers in dozens of countries across the globe.) Genetic testing should be given for the purpose of preparation and decision making, not as a tool for predicting the quality of a child's life.

The right to legal and safe abortion is a core element of American feminism and the struggle for women's rights. This puts me in a strange position. When I think about this issue, I feel my very existence questioned. As a disabled woman, I have been told flat out, "I'd rather be dead than be like you." Even the Dalai Lama has said that aborting a fetus with a disability is understandable. How do I begin to hold this contradiction in my mind? That I am a valid, beautiful human being—as are all my friends, some of whom have much severer impairments—and that I also support women's right to choose, a right that logically must extend to a woman who ends a pregnancy because of the prospect of an extra finger? I don't know the answer, but somehow, I believe the treatment I received as a disabled woman who chose to conceive—the disrespect, the testing, the constant questioning of my capacity to give birth and to be a mother—and my response to it fit into this equation.

Some days, I look at my son, who is now 14, and I want to pull my hair out. OK, most days. Here I am tempted to compile a list of the ways he makes my life difficult and tedious. But that list is unnecessary. That's not because my son is perfect, but because he's perfect to me. Because I love the person he has become, not the person I wish him to be.

If You're in a Wheelchair, Segregation Lives

LUTICHA DOUCETTE

IN 2016, THE FORMER CHIEF OF THE SANTA FE, N.M., POLICE DEPARTMENT, Donald Grady II, said something that stuck with me. "There's a thing that we call freedom of movement," he said in an interview with The Atlantic, "which is really revered in this country—that we should have the right to move freely without impingement from the police simply because." He was speaking as both a black man and a police officer about the ways racial discrimination can limit a basic right. But I related to this on more than one level.

As a black woman with incomplete quadriplegia and chronic pain, and as a full-time manual wheelchair user, my own ability to move freely is frequently restricted. Too often, both the lack of accessibility in public spaces and the ingrained ableism of many nondisabled people bar my way.

Let's say I want to go out to dinner downtown. Even if I can enter an establishment—which I often can't—very rarely is the accessible seating in a visible place, if it is there at all. Once inside, I am often relegated to a corner, the aisle, a back room. In brew pubs with high tables and high chairs, trying to have conversations at eye level with other people's crotches while nursing my beer leads me to feel less like an adult and more like Oliver Twist. No one wants to try the new hot spot in town and then be seated at the kids' table.

If I arrive somewhere by myself, I am often greeted with shock when I make clear that I have no caregiver with me. If I am with a companion—a nondisabled friend or a date—it is assumed that this person is my caregiver. Sometimes it seems that people believe accessibility is having your own chaperone who goes and asks for the accessible entrance.

These are just a few variations on the sort of ableism that people with physical conditions like mine face every day. Ableism is at work when disability is not an inclusive part of the design process, where the space flows and is welcoming to all bodies. Instead, accommodations are tacked on haphazardly, leading to hostile and hard-to-navigate spaces. With the passage of the Americans With Disabilities Act in 1990—which sets standards of compliance for buildings in public spaces—progress has been made, but inclusive thinking and design are still the exception, not the norm.

Today, segregation and limiting the movement of disabled persons in public spaces is commonplace and accepted. Even in our nation's capital, I have to use the back entrance at the National Gallery of Art. As a black woman I am keenly aware of the irony of being ushered through back ways, sketchy hallways, side entrances and kitchens to enter restaurants, bars and other establishments. My favorite bar up the street has its accessible entrance down an alley, with a steep ramp that leads to a door in the bowels of the building. There's no signage, no security cameras, and I once saw a bloody towel covering the fire alarm. At another local restaurant, I have to enter from a side door, through the kitchen and then to the dining room. It is a running joke with my friends that if the accessible entrance is not up front, you're going to end up needing a map to find your way through.

Some aspects of this situation, though, are too painful to joke about. Much of what people with disabilities like mine must suffer conjures the historically painful specter of racial segregation. Even at my job, where I work for the city as a researcher in a government building, there is an entrance with a double doorway for those walking in, then next to it, hidden around a pillar, a sliding door for wheelchair users. The other exterior doors have stairs leading up to them. My employer did a wonderful job in doing a walk-through with me to identify ways to solve the problem, but this raises a key point: The building was built in a time when people with disabilities were almost entirely hidden from society, and architects did not consider how such a person would use the building. This makes retrofitting an even bigger challenge. All this eerily mirrors the segregation of blacks in the workplace, where separate doors were not unusual. We need to be just as vigilant about disability inclusion as we are about racial inclusion.

In the social justice space, ableism would be categorized as a macroaggression. Disability comes with its own unique challenges and trials, but the inability to engage with, and move freely through, our communities, or not being able to easily visit friends' and relatives' homes—and the social isolation that follows—because inclusive design is so uncommon, is a gross violation of our rights and is detrimental to our health.

Our freedom of movement is hindered in other ways. *How* we move as disabled people often leads to poor encounters with the police. We are often taken for drunks, our caregivers are harmed, or even shot; we are perceived as threats and beaten when trying to communicate in sign language, or worse, killed. In March, a report published by the Ruderman Family Foundation highlighted that half of police shootings have involved a disabled person. They were also people of color. Yet these deaths are rarely spoken of in the context of the person's disability.

To make things worse, the intersection of race, poverty and disability is often ignored. Black Lives Matter has come under much deserved criticism by black and Latinx disability rights activists for lack of inclusion in their "woke" spaces. We cannot be fully woke if we refuse to acknowledge our disabled brothers and sisters. My city has some of the highest poverty rates for minorities and for the disabled. A recent study ranked Rochester 147th out of 150 American cities in a list of best and worst places to live if you are disabled. Yet, those in poverty who are disabled live in the highest-poverty census tracts, have very low education levels, no access to jobs and a shortage of affordable, accessible housing, and lack the resources to move within their communities, which have poor transportation options. They very rarely have the opportunity to live somewhere else, nor can they fully engage with the myriad initiatives designed to lift people out of poverty.

For me, freedom of movement also encompasses the ability to move in environments without people coming up to me and touching me or invading my personal space. Black women know the violating feeling when someone decides to touch our hair without permission as we go about our daily lives. Disability adds another layer to it. A poignant moment was during prep for an M.R.I. My hair was ripped out by a white female technician because she was "curious about its softness." My blackness was singled out and my disability used against me. She took a moment where I was vulnerable and exploited that.

But these body-autonomy violations are a regular occurrence. People push my chair without asking, and often in the wrong direction, and shove me in the back as a way of "helping" me propel my chair—my movement and autonomy are constantly being challenged. And just as black men experience people moving to the other side of the street or white women clutching their purses on the assumption that they are a threat, I too experience people jumping out of the way or pulling their children to them in fear as they loudly proclaim that they don't want to be hit by a wheelchair, even when I'm several feet from them. To be treated as something to avoid but also something to be touched at will creates an odd juxtaposition that is unique to the black disabled experience.

Navigating the world as a black woman is difficult, but I refuse to give up the fight to dismantle structural racism and structural ableism. At the core of the civil rights movement, Black Lives Matter and the disability rights movement is the idea of autonomy and agency over one's life. We are fighting for the right to not be judged based on external sets of unrealistic expectations. The rights afforded to us in the Constitution are not fully granted to us if we are constantly obstructed by structural biases. To that end, I would paraphrase Chief Grady's definition to be even more inclusive: We should have the right to move freely without impingement from *anyone or anything*. Simply because.

My Medicaid, My Life

ALICE WONG

I AM A MEDICAID WELFARE QUEEN. WHEN REPUBLICANS TALK ABOUT safety net programs like Medicaid, Social Security and food stamps, they evoke images of people like me gabbing on their smartphones, eating steak and watching TV from the comfort of home. Political rhetoric and media coverage paints us as unmotivated and undeserving individuals, passive consumers of taxpayer dollars who are out to "game the system," taking resources away from hard-working people.

The reality of being a disabled person on Medicaid is far more complex and nuanced. Many people do not even know the difference between Medicaid and Medicare and simply consider them "entitlement programs," as if tax breaks and corporate subsidies aren't entitlements by another name. Medicaid is more than a health care program. It is a life-giving program.

Like the thousands of people sharing their stories at town halls about how the Affordable Care Act saved their lives, I am sharing my Medicaid story to illustrate its value and the potential consequences of "reform."

I am an Asian-American woman with a disability and a daughter of immigrants. When I turned 18, my dad told me that I needed to make an appointment at the county office and apply for Medicaid. Living in an affluent suburb of Indianapolis, I was indignant. Medicaid was for "those people," the "indigent." I learned that my parents paid exorbitant monthly premiums for my health care. Only one company in our state would cover me because of my preexisting condition (spinal muscular atrophy, a congenital motor neuron disease). I had no idea of the financial pressure placed on our family for basic health insurance because of my disability.

I graduated from high school in 1992, two years after the Americans With Disabilities Act was passed. Learning about disability history and realizing I was a member of a protected class encouraged me to imagine and create the life that I want. Once I got over myself and realized I had a right to Medicaid, it made a difference immediately.

I began to receive several hours a week of services to help me with personal care. When I went away to college I was able to hire attendants and live independently for the first time. It was an exhilarating taste of freedom that showed me a glimpse of what was possible. Before Medicaid, my family members, including my siblings, provided all of my care, including bathing, dressing and toileting. Now I had choices and the basic human right of self-determination.

Unfortunately, Indiana made cuts to Medicaid the following year that resulted in fewer hours of services. Our family couldn't manage both tuition and private pay for personal care, so I made the heartbreaking decision to leave the school I loved and move back home.

As I commuted to a school nearby, I learned about the activism by disabled people that led to expanded accessibility and services across the country, California in particular. Moving to San Francisco for graduate school in the late 1990s afforded me the privilege of being in a state with a program that allows me to direct my own personal care services, including hiring and training my attendants. This program, In-Home Supportive Services, is funded by a combination of local, state and federal funds. Without it, I wouldn't have been able to go to school, work or volunteer.

By no means is it fun or easy receiving Medicaid. I follow strict eligibility rules and guidelines. I've been able to work as a researcher thanks to a state Medicaid Working Disabled Program where I can maintain eligibility by paying monthly premiums. Over time, my disability progressed and I needed substantial care that would normally take place in an institution if I didn't have any help. I became eligible for additional hours of service through a Medicaid waiver so that I could remain in the community and stay out of a nursing home, at a considerable savings cost for the entire system.

When you are disabled and rely on public services and programs, you face vulnerability every day. This vulnerability is felt in my bones and my relationship with the state. Fluctuations in the economy and politics determine whether my attendants will receive a living wage and whether I'll have enough services to subsist rather than thrive. The fragility and weakness of my body, I can handle. The fragility of the safety net is something I fear and worry about constantly.

Although the American Health Care Act—the Republican attempt to replace the Obama administration's Affordable Care Act—failed, the assault on poor, disabled, sick and older people continues in other forms. The Centers for Medicaid and Medicare Services can weaken regulations, place limits on the services states provide without legislation and add new work requirements. States can request block grants and changes to eligibility and regulations from the federal government directly. Block grants and per capita limits will force states to reduce or eliminate services to make up the difference from the federal government, affecting millions of people.

"Program flexibility" is code for the decimation of Medicaid that will put lives like mine at risk. Some people with disabilities may have to live in nursing homes if community-based services wither away under this flexibility and reform. We cannot disappear again after a history of segregation and institutionalization. When Republicans talk about freedom and choice, they don't realize that Medicaid gives those very things to people with disabilities.

March 2017 marked my 25th year of being a recipient of Medicaid. When I was young, I felt shame and embarrassment at being one of "those people" on benefits. Today I am unapologetically disabled and a fully engaged member of society. None of that would be possible without Medicaid.

Every day I resist forces that label me as the Other or a scapegoat for society's problems. With the disability community, I share our stories and speak out against threats to our future by using my privilege and tools such as social media. I hope my story will continue for decades to come.

You Are Special! Now Stop Being Different

JONATHAN MOONEY

LET ME TELL YOU ABOUT MY RELATIONSHIP WITH THE SCHOOL DESK. From my first day at Penny Camp Elementary School in 1982, it was fraught.

This is how it went down: Five seconds into class, the foot starts bouncing; 10 seconds in, both feet; 15 seconds, I bust out the drums! After a few minutes, it's all over. I'm trying to put my leg behind my neck. No, that desk and I didn't get along. For some kids it was just school furniture, but for me it was a form of enhanced interrogation that would have made Dick Cheney smile.

I was shamed for not sitting still. Shamed at home at the dinner table with my dad, where I heard "Stop it stop it stop it what is wrong with you?" And I was shamed in school. I had a second-grade teacher, Ms. C—I have had many gifted teachers in my life, for which I am grateful, but Ms. C wasn't one. When my foot was bouncing, she would stop class, point at me and say at the top of her lungs, "Jonathan, what is your problem?"

Sitting still was hard enough, but I also struggled with reading and was placed in the "dumb" group. Teachers didn't actually call us the "dumb" group, but let's be real: Everyone knew which group was the "smart" group and which wasn't—my school had the California Condors, the Blackbirds, the Bluebirds, and then over in the annex trailer building, the Sparrows. I spent the day reading "See Spot Run" while the Condors were probably finishing up "War and Peace."

Joking aside, no matter what the reading groups were named, kids knew their place on the intelligence bell curve. "See Spot Run" is not a bad book. Nice narrative structure. Good moral tale. But I didn't want to be caught dead with "Spot" when I was 10 years old. So as I headed across the room to find my reading group, "Spot" went in my backpack, under my shirt, because as I walked by the other kids the taunts would start: "Jonathan, go back to the dumb reading group."

Reading out loud in class was a special kind of hell. I couldn't focus on the page and would excuse myself and hide in the bathroom, hoping I would miss my turn. I never did. Those 10 minutes in front of the class fumbling and stammering gave me an extra helping of humiliation and shame.

By the third grade I had progressed from being one of "those kids" to being the "special ed." kid. I was found to have multiple language-based learning disabilities and attention deficit disorder. When the educational psychologist broke the news to my mom and me, it was as if someone had died. Tissues on the table. Hushed tones. Mirrors covered. Sat shiva for the death of my normality. The tragedy of my problem wasn't lost on me, even at 8 years old. People thought something was wrong with me, and I knew it.

Wearing this label, I found myself in a variety of settings focused primarily on remediating my deficits. Ground zero was spelling. Every Friday was spelling test day. Every day leading up to spelling test day was remediation day. Monday I was drawing my spelling words in the sand. Tuesday I would build them with blocks. Wednesday, flash cards. And Thursday I would do interpretive dance to get those words into my head. Friday? I'd fail the test, every time. I was the round peg that needed to be squared, a revenue stream for the remediation industrial complex; I spent hours a day being fixed.

I was turned into a "patient" who needed treatment rather than a human being with differences to be empowered. Fixing takes its toll. My self-image plummeted. I had a great teacher named Mr. R who asked me to describe myself. I told him I was the "stupid" kid. I gave up hope.

In the middle of sixth grade my parents withdrew me from Penny Camp, and after trying out other options, I dropped out of school. I struggled with severe anxiety and depression at age 10.

I survived this time in my life because of my mom. On a good day, Colleen Mooney, on her tiptoes, is 5 foot 1. She barely graduated from high school and never went to college. She raised my brother and two sisters on welfare in San Francisco. She also has, let's just say, an interesting voice and vocabulary. She sounds like Mickey Mouse and she curses like a truck driver. So you can imagine when I was having a hard time in school, if you were a principal or a teacher doing wrong by her son, you did not want her in your office. But she often was. She knew in her heart that her child wasn't broken and didn't need to be fixed.

My mom was right. When I think back on my school experience, I realize it wasn't the ADD or the dyslexia that disabled me. I'm not naïve about the bad stuff that comes with my brain. I struggle with executive functioning and organization, I have explored the feasibility of stapling my car keys to my forehead, and I spell at a third-grade level. But guess what? Good things come with this brain.

Research shows that learning and attention differences correlate with enhanced problem solving, creativity and entrepreneurship. What disabled me were limitations not in myself but in the environment: the passive learning experience where students sit at a desk most of the day; a narrow definition of intelligence conflated with reading and other right-brain skills; and a medicalization of differences that reduced my brain to a set of deficits and ignored the strengths that go hand in hand with many brain differences.

I've come to believe that I did not *have* a disability, as it is common to say, but *experienced* disability in environments that could not accommodate and embrace my differences. Ability/disability is not a fact in the world but a social construct, what Michel Foucault called a "transactional reality" created by public policy, professional power and everything in between. All of us, even the so-called normal, move in and out of states of ability and disability every day. It's our strengths, weaknesses, eccentricities and differences that define our humanity.

As a society, America has the rhetoric of differences down. On the first day of kindergarten we are told that we are all special. But then the bell rings and that message changes: Now sit down, keep quiet and do what everyone else is doing. They tell you what to learn, when to learn and how to learn. *We love the individual; now stop being different.*

I never did get "fixed." The rest of my education was up and down. I struggled in cookie-cutter classes and thrived when teachers accommodated my learning differences. My mom told me if I survived high school, college and life would be better. She was right.

In the fall of 1997, after two years at Loyola Marymount University, where my learning differences were fully accommodated, I transferred to Brown University, where I graduated with an honors degree in English literature. I still can't spell or sit still, but I now use support and technology to mitigate my weakness and build a life on my strengths. I don't feel stupid anymore and I know that I—and others like me—can live good lives despite these challenges.

A fundamental battleground for every civil rights movement has been the rejection of the idea that you're the problem and a demand for cultural and systemic change. Whether one believes that people like me are disabled or persons with a disability, or simply different, we all require the same things: schools, workplaces and communities that are inclusive of the diversity of human minds and bodies. We have to fight for every person's right to be different.

Brain Injury and the Civil Right We Don't Think About

JOSEPH J. FINS

THE LAST TIME I SAW MARGARET WORTHEN WAS IN NOVEMBER 2012. She was in New York participating in a study of patients with severe brain injury. As soon as I walked into her room, I knew something had changed. She was still immobile, but she noticed my presence, was more attentive and engaged. And there was something else: She at times was able to use her left eye to answer simple yes or no questions. That morning, she seemed to relish her newfound fluency. She responded with verve, as if the determined downward swoop of her eye could signal an exclamation point.

Communicating with one eye may not seem like much, but it was something to behold. Maggie, as she was known, had suffered a complex stroke six years earlier, during her senior year at Smith College, that involved areas deep in her brain. She had been thought to be in the "vegetative state"—the term commonly used to define the unconscious brain state most of us associate with the right to die movement and the legacies of Karen Ann Quinlan, Nancy Cruzan and Terri Schiavo.

Later, Maggie was found to be in the "minimally conscious state"—a term medically formalized in 2002. Unlike vegetative patients, those in MCS *are* conscious. They demonstrate intention, attention and memory. They may reach for a cup, say their name and notice you when you walk into their room. The problem is that these actions may be rare and intermittent, so when family members who witnessed them share their observations with staff members, they are often attributed to a family's wishful thinking.

This may be true in individual cases. But often it is just part and parcel of the biology of MCS. Indeed, at least one study indicated an alarming rate of misdiagnosis: It found that 41 percent of patients with traumatic brain injury who were in chronic care and thought to be in the vegetative state were in fact in MCS.

If not for the astute observations of her Boston neurologist, Maggie, too, would have been misdiagnosed in perpetuity. But instead, she was expressing herself one blink at a time. For a young woman who had been thought permanently unconscious, this was truly a heroic accomplishment.

Maggie's mother, Nancy, who gave me permission to tell her family's story in my book, "Rights Come to Mind: Brain Injury, Ethics and the Struggle for Consciousness," never thought this would be how her daughter's life would turn out. She had other expectations for her beautiful daughter, who studied Spanish, played Frisbee and aspired to be a veterinarian.

Still, Nancy and Maggie made a life together after the stroke. And it was OK. Nancy was grateful that Maggie had learned to communicate, while wishing she could do more than move that one eye. Still, she told me, it seemed like it was "enough to have a life, even a small life." Maggie had things that many people didn't have, she said—relationships, friends and family who loved her.

In the end, Nancy arrived at a sort of acceptance: "So, I don't know. But I think a small life is OK."

We cannot know whether it was OK for Maggie. But the rudimentary communication channel established with her left eye was the start of a way to know what she might have thought. That we cannot yet know for sure did not mean that she had no preferences or wishes. Indeed the goal of those of us who do this work is to find out and try to provide these patients with the chance to again express their agency.

Maggie's case—her "small life"—became very consequential

when my colleagues at Weill Cornell Medicine published a paper in December 2016 in the journal Science Translational Medicine revealing what had happened within her brain following her injury. During the recovery of her ability to communicate, Maggie's brain essentially rewired over a period of years.

Using magnetic resonance imaging, Daniel J. Thengone, a graduate student, and colleagues in the Laboratory of Cognitive Neuromodulation, led by Dr. Nicholas D. Schiff, were able to demonstrate a strengthening of structural and functional reconnections across the two hemispheres emanating from Broca's area, the region in the frontal lobe responsible for speech. It showed, remarkably, that even a grievously injured brain could heal itself. It appeared to do so by a process bearing a strong resemblance to typical brain development. The ongoing reorganization of connections among neurons is a reprise of how the developing brain gets its start.

As notable as these findings were, they did not stem from a high tech or costly intervention. Instead, they were the byproduct of a mother's love, speech therapy and a simple eye-tracking device that cost about $30. It was Freud's "talking cure" in a modern guise, and no less significant for our understanding of resilience and the importance of interpersonal engagement.

Yet, access to care is strained for this population. Utilization reviewers and insurance benefit companies will deny access to rehabilitation to many individuals when they leave the hospital because they are deemed not yet ready for rehabilitation. But when nearly half of those who could participate are misdiagnosed as vegetative when they are actually minimally conscious, this vulnerable group is further marginalized. Organizations like the American College of Rehabilitation Medicine have been calling for a comprehensive evaluation of patients after hospital discharge so that misdiagnosis can be prevented and those who might be helped can get the rehabilitation they need.

Even those lucky few who do get rehabilitation and are not shunted off to what is euphemistically called "custodial care" get too little time. Most rehab stays are six weeks or less. But if the brain recovers through a slow process similar to development, why do we provide—and only to those lucky enough to receive it—just a few hours of rehabilitation a week for six weeks? It would be akin to sending your third grader to school for half-days of classes for a month or two and telling them that they are now on their own. Now that we know that it takes years for the developing brain to learn and mature, a similar commitment to the recovering injured brain now seems indicated.

If we reconceived rehabilitation as education, no one would graduate after a six-week course of care. Instead, we would promote lifelong learning as a means to achieve a recovered life. If there is a legal obligation to educate the developing brain, should there not be a correlative responsibility to those whose brains are in a process of redevelopment and recovery?

These are radical propositions at a time of fiscal scarcity and serious debate about the fate of Obamacare and health care reform. Understood this way, one might see the surrounding politics as untenable and reasonably seek to spend resources elsewhere. But it would be a mistake to view our responsibilities so narrowly. What is at stake here is more than a simple insurance question or access to care. It is a more fundamental question of basic civil rights, leaving conscious individuals isolated and abandoned.

Tragically, the most fundamental rights have been denied patients in the minimally conscious state.

Take pain control, for example. When a minimally conscious patient is mistakenly diagnosed as vegetative and thus thought insensate, they may not receive analgesic pain management or anesthesia for medical procedures. If this occurs, they are incredibly vulnerable—unable to communicate, and thus unable to cry out in pain. This error of omission constitutes a disrespect for personhood that should be beyond the pale in any civilized society.

Of course, we can address this by better diagnostic assessments of a patient's brain state, to differentiate the minimally conscious from the permanently unconscious patient. But we can do something more. We can work to restore the patients' own voices, so that they can tell us whether they are in pain, and remind us that they are in the room. They remain members of the human community even though society has segregated them in chronic care.

I use the verb "segregated" deliberately, to invoke a time when separate but equal was the law. In the wake of legal advances like the Americans with Disabilities Act and the United Nations Convention on the Rights of the Disabled, which call for the integration of people with disabilities into civil society, how is the pervasive segregation of this population justified?

Part of the problem is that when these laws were written, the notion of reintegration was focused on physical mobility—the ramp on the side walk and the accessible workplace. It wasn't about people whose means of integration required something more than a ramp. For minimally conscious patients, the ramp is the restoration of functional communication, which makes reintegration into its cognate—community—possible. When we restore voice to these patients we bring them back into the room and the conversation.

To accomplish this we must consider the basic relationship between these individuals and the state, and their civil rights as citizens. Legal protections have eluded this population precisely because they have been disenfranchised by their injury. They have fallen outside the scope of legal protections and been subject to abuse and neglect.

This is the civil rights issue most of us never thought about. But the long arc of justice is sometimes refracted through scientific discovery and medical advances.

I often speak to university students brought up in the era of LGBTQ rights who can't understand how my generation did not appreciate that people could love those they chose to love. They find it incomprehensible that this almost self-evident right had eluded earlier generations. I caution against smugness, suggesting that their own children may well ask them how they allowed society to ignore conscious individuals and deprive them of *their* rights.

We now can anticipate that there are large numbers of people like Maggie, who have the potential to communicate but are sequestered—indeed, segregated—in chronic care, isolated and abandoned by society. Some could be identified with proper screening and coaxed back through rehabilitation and emerging treatments. Now that we know this, we can't look away.

Sadly, it is too late for Maggie, who died on Aug. 2, 2015. But it's not for others who linger in the isolation of their own heads waiting for a chance to talk with you and exercise their newly found rights. No doubt, it will be an interesting conversation.

II

BELONGING

I Don't Want to Be "Inspiring"

JOHN ALTMANN

ONE OF MY MOST MEMORABLE MOMENTS IN HIGH SCHOOL CAME DURING my freshman year. A motivational speaker was addressing us in a huge assembly. I was seated with one of my best friends at the front of the auditorium, and the whole group was having an amazing time. The speaker was charismatic, exhibited a warm, jovial disposition and a wonderful sense of humor. I was smiling and laughing with the rest of the group. But at the end of the assembly, my friend and I were singled out by the speaker, who said something that people with disabilities hear often—that because I got around on crutches and she with a scooter, we were "inspiring."

In that moment my personal characteristics, the people I love, the interests I pursue and the beliefs I hold became moot, and the fact that I have cerebral palsy and use crutches to walk became the entirety of who John Altmann is and what he is about.

When I tried expressing my anger to people, I felt disconnected from them. They assured me the speaker was just being nice; some insisted he was just telling the truth. That what I did every day *was* inspiring. I grew tired trying to convince them that I shouldn't be a source of inspiration for anyone simply because I live my life as I know it just like everyone else.

The friend who I sat with at the assembly got it. Our frustration, while a foreign language to all of our able-bodied friends, arose from a deeper desire that we shared. We wanted to be more than our disabilities, to overcome them and forge an identity apart from them. But an able-bodied world makes it hard to find this sort of fulfillment. And it often does so with even the best of intentions.

Case in point: In January a story made the rounds about an undefeated wrestler who let his opponent, who happened to have Down syndrome, win a match. Most people praised the athlete for being selfless and a class act. A reporter at CNN wrote, "A high school wrestling star gave up a shot at going undefeated this year, but some people think he had the perfect season." I didn't see it that way.

Wrestling is an activity predicated upon a specific kind of athletic acumen and is governed by its own set of rules. When the undefeated wrestler let the opponent with Down syndrome win, the nature of the environment was fundamentally altered. The wrestling mat, which is meant to be a site for athletes to exhibit their physical prowess and to find out in the end who the superior wrestler is, became instead another site of segregation.

I don't mean to say the wrestler had malicious intent; it's obvious that his heart was in the right place, but his actions, and more significantly society's subsequent reaction to them, reinforced the stigma that the disabled body is one in need of our sympathy and charity. In that moment the wrestler's identity was disregarded and his disability took center stage. However well intentioned, the able-bodied wrestler chose segregation by laying down for his opponent rather than giving him his best. His sympathy became toxic.

This is just a symptom of a much larger problem. Society, on an institutional level, consistently opts for its own more profound types of segregation. In Britain, for instance, welfare reforms caused 14,000 disabled citizens to lose the mobility cars they use to function and to go about their lives. Here in the United States, one of the most common and widespread problems for people with disabilities is unemployment, with only about 40 percent of disabled people employed as of 2010, about half the rate of nondisabled people. These problems can be linked with the inaccessibility disabled students usually encounter in colleges and other spheres of civil society.

Much like the Civil Rights Act for African-Americans, the Americans With Disabilities Act, while a revolutionary piece of legislation at the time of its passage, was not a magic wand we could wave to dismantle these transgressions against disabled people, or reform the system that supports them.

Disabled people cannot be expected to forge an identity beyond their disability or to diminish the impact that their disability has on them personally, psychologically or emotionally when they are deprived of the very extensions of their bodies that allow them to engage in the world, and when this very engagement is faced with exclusion. When a college, a business or any sphere of civil society refuses the expenditure on accommodation of a disabled person, and when a government actively deprives disabled people of what they need to live, they're effectively saying that what we are outside of our disabilities and what we wish to become in spite of them doesn't matter.

I want a world that is so accessible, where technology and medicine become so advanced, that all disabled people get the chance to opt out of their disability. I want a world where the social relations I forge with those who are able-bodied are not predicated on my disability.

As the philosopher of disability Joel Michael Reynolds has said, the world is essentially disabled. Deprive a man of an elevator or a flight of stairs, and could he make it from the first floor to the second? He couldn't, and it would be absurd to accentuate this inability to the point where it became all the man was. So too is it absurd to boil me down to my needing crutches to traverse the world. I am John Altmann, I am not my cerebral palsy. When this becomes common sense to the world, then I will have effectively escaped my disability, even though I will always use my crutches to do so.

The Deaf Body in Public Space

RACHEL KOLB

"IT'S RUDE TO POINT," MY FRIEND TOLD ME FROM ACROSS THE ELEMENTARY-school cafeteria table. I grasped her words as I read them off her lips. She stared at my index finger, which I held raised in midair, gesturing toward a mutual classmate. "My mom said so."

I was 6 or 7 years old, but I remember stopping with a jolt. Something inside me froze, too, went suddenly cold.

"I'm signing," I said out loud. "That's not rude."

As the only deaf student in my elementary school, I had already stumbled across the challenges of straddling two languages and two modes of communication. My family was hearing, but they still empowered me by using both English and sign language at home.

A sign language interpreter accompanied me throughout the day at school, and my teachers created a welcoming environment for me to learn, but finding a place to belong with kids my own age often felt more difficult. I tried to speak to them, and occasionally they reciprocated the effort by learning some basic signs. But usually I felt separate.

I went home that day and asked my mother about what my friend had said. "Don't worry," my mother said, "she doesn't know the social rules are different with signing. You aren't being rude." With that, matter-of-fact as always, she brought the conversation to an end. But I still felt a lingering self-consciousness, entirely novel and difficult to shake.

This was perhaps the first time I realized that other people could see me as obtrusive, as taking up too much space, when I was simply communicating just as I was.

When I reflect on this memory two decades later, I recognize how my childhood friend, whom at the time I had found to be so accusatory, had really gaped at me with a sort of wonder. My signing challenged the rules of social conduct she'd absorbed from adults, and to her I must have seemed ignorant or radically rebellious, or perhaps both. But pointing was a truly fundamental act for me; it was how I expressed what my grown-up scholarly self would call *relationality*—the idea of being in the world in relation to others. Through sign language, a properly poised finger allowed me to say *you* and *me* and *he* and *she* and *they*. If I did not point, how could I make a human connection?

Many years later, when I was in graduate school, another conversation with a friend made an impression on me. We were in a cafe having lunch; she was one of those rare friends who had started learning sign language solely to communicate with me. That day over lunch we forfeited spoken English, which we typically used to talk with each other, and practiced conversing with our hands and our facial expressions. I felt a touch of exhilaration; she was putting aside her conventional, ingrained hearingness and coming to meet me in my visual world.

But after a few minutes, my usually bold, unself-conscious friend stopped. She chuckled and shrugged a little, and said, "I feel like everyone here is *looking at us*."

I glanced around the small cafe, at all the hearing people sitting at their tables. Indeed, some had craned their necks to look at our movements, but this was behavior I'd long ago ceased to notice. "Yeah," I signed back, bluntly. "That often happens."

My friend smiled. A moment later, we started conversing again, and I think then she understood: *This* is what it can be like to occupy a signing body.

To use sign language, to embrace it in non-signing public spaces, one must sometimes push against ideas of having committed a gross indiscretion. These notions, I confess, haunted my relationship with my body for years after my childhood friend told me not to point. How obvious signing was, how indiscreet in the "conventional" sense: what I was pointing at, my lively facial expressions, my sense of physical restraint! I was already shy as a child, reluctant to put myself on display. So for a while I felt embarrassed, but then learned not to be. This happened out of necessity, out of self-acceptance and, frankly, joy in my own signing body, but for other nonnative signers it happens out of choice. As several other hearing friends have told me since, when they sign with me in public they feel rather conspicuous. "Should I do this?" they ask me. "Is it too much?"

Too much: To me these words succinctly articulate the taboos that can linger about bodily expressiveness. Hearing culture presents us with ideals of speaking with good elocution, restraint and self-control. Now, I admit, I see these ideals as visually impoverished, inaccessible and uninteresting: They produce spaces full of immobile talking heads, disembodied sound and visual inattentiveness. Those qualities become the optical equivalent of speaking in a monotone. As much as I also enjoy spoken words, allowing my body to speak for itself feels, simply, more real. Even if that means signing is sometimes read as a visual spectacle.

My hearing friends, who have often never had to cope with being looked at, can struggle the most with this sense of spectacle. When they learn to sign with me—and there are still too few who *really* learn—they must overcome these cultural taboos about excessive movement, pointing and gesture. Over the years, I have kept a mental list of the comments they make at the beginning stages.

"I don't know what to do with my hands. It's like I've just discovered I have them."

"Are you sure it's OK to point? At *him*?"

"I *am* trying to be more expressive. My face just feels like it can't."

"That feels weird."

"How do your eyes take in so much information, so fast?"

And finally: "I feel self-conscious. I feel like you are looking at me."

Yes, I want to tell people who regale me with that last comment. Yes, I am looking at you, because what would the point be otherwise?

Over time, I hope that the direct gaze comes to feel as affirming to my hearing companions as it does to me. When I sign, when I use my body to communicate, it indeed elicits a different state of mind, one that invites and guides the physical gaze, but this need not feel discomforting or unwelcome. On the contrary: Looking at me, at my body and everything it says, shows me that you are paying attention. We meet each other in the midst of this physical and linguistic self-expression, and our connection surpasses a disembodied voice and expands to include our entire beings. Right here, looking back at you, I feel like I have made contact.

My "Orphan Disease" Has Given Me a New Family

ROSEMARIE GARLAND-THOMSON

THE MEMBERS OF MY FAMILY SHARE A NUMBER OF TRAITS, BUT NOT one of them looks quite like me.

Many of us have the same sturdy physique, blue eyes, fine Northern European hair and skin that should never see bright sun. I look pretty much like that except for one very unusual characteristic. I was born with asymmetrical, atypical hands and forearms into a world where symmetry and typicality are the marks of good looks and proper function. In fact, I am so unusual that in the half century of my lifetime, I have encountered only one other person who looks precisely like me. In other words, I'm rare.

I recently learned that I am distinguished in this way because I have a rare genetic condition—complex syndactyly. Before I learned this, no medical doctor had ever presented a diagnosis more helpful than a shrug.

Before being able to identify and give a name to what I have, I was subject to plenty of unsavory terms: "freak of nature," "funny-looking kid," "deformed," "birth anomaly," "sporadic limb deficiency." The most disagreeable and persistent was "birth defect," the unfortunate outcome of whatever sin or defilement could be guessed at or imagined—alcohol consumption, pollution, environmental contamination. With no impressive diagnosis to offer to the perpetual query about "what happened" to me, I usually resorted to, "I was born that way."

I'm glad to now have a "rare genetic condition" instead of a "birth defect." Anything "rare" has prestige, suggesting something sought after and prized by important collectors, archaeologists or scientists. Indeed, so exceptional is my way of being that fewer than one in 90,000 people are enough like me to receive the same diagnosis. It's a bit like winning the lottery.

Before decades of scientific work gave us the genome map in 2003, our ways to explain unexpected human variation were limited. People like me were inexplicable. As often happens with the inexplicable, supernatural and superstitious reasoning rushed in. Mother-blaming and divine retribution were prominent. Any social code violation or mortal sins or erotic thoughts were thought to produce a disabled child.

Modern versions of this superstition haunt the mothers of congenitally disabled children; they experience corrosive guilt about exposure to toxins ranging from face cream and nail polish, alcohol and cigarettes, to thalidomide and the BPA in our plastic bottles. People with disabilities were then and are now taken as cautions or warnings of bad things past or future, canaries in the coal mine of human existence.

But things have changed. "Rare" is now an inflection in my personal dignity tool kit, a status upgrade. Even "syndrome" has an air of sophistication, an augmentation rather than the lessening that "deficit" or "defect" brings. It's something you *have* instead of something you *don't have*. More important, my form is not a mistake, some random whack from a menacing outside world. My shape is intentional, manifesting deliberately from some mysterious purpose at the very core of my being. Evolution's purposive caprice, some inexplicable force beyond our puny human imagination, is trying out a new design.

Today, identifying genetic diseases is a growth industry, powered by scientific-research funding and lucrative commercial interests. With testing available everywhere now, from private companies to clinics, people whose genetic diseases have been identified are an increasing population. All of us, it turns out, are carriers for at least eight to 10 common, significant genetic diseases and even more rare, enigmatic conditions.

What this tells us is that we are all related to one another through a system of genetic lineage that almost no one understood until recently. These genetic kinship circles are expanding and connecting us through networks of recessive, dominant and autosomal genes; mitochondrial DNA; and complex interactions with the environment that shape how genes express themselves as we develop. Medical science has discovered more than 7,000 genetic diseases, and new ones emerge every day.

People in my world of disability pride and advocacy sometimes call themselves by tribal names such as "a thalidomide" or "a polio" or even "crips." Our new genetic identities now yield more complex affinities. Rare genetic conditions are also called "orphan diseases." Now that I have an orphan disease instead of a birth defect, I'm no longer an orphan but instead newly a member of several distinctive tribes, a heretofore hidden web of kinship and clan affiliations. Resemblances are crucial to kinship, whether familial, tribal or ethnic. What we look like tells us and other people to whom we belong. Our distinctive traits gather us in kinship networks that often provide us with alternative families of mutual care and support.

In a recent conversation about Crispr, the newest genetic editing tool, the geneticist and Nobel laureate Mario R. Capecchi told me, "The purpose of evolution is to anticipate the unexpected." Random genetic variation is what moves evolution forward, yielding new forms that are fresh solutions to changing environments both natural and human designed.

The short span of human life and imagination limits our capacities to anticipate the unexpected. Ways of being that meet the demands of human life as we live it here and now may not serve our distant descendants so well. Characteristics we think of as intelligence, strength, vision, uprightness, dexterity, body mass or whiteness will outlive their usefulness, morphing from advantages to disadvantages, counterintuitive though that seems today, especially perhaps to those who have those valued traits and benefit from them.

Capecchi's framing of evolution's purpose as anticipating the unexpected can give us progressive perceptions about living with disabilities and stand as a caution against hubris and narcissism in our aspirations to shape our human communities according to the traits valued by the majority.

People with disabilities are the unexpected made flesh. The challenges of living in a world not built for us are occasions for resourcefulness and adaptability, especially for those of us who start out disabled early in life. We are innovators, early adopters, expert users and technology hackers as we respond to the adversity that the built and natural environments present us.

We don't know which human variations will be advantages and which will be disadvantages in the long arc of our struggle to prevail in an ever-changing environment. My blind friend with excellent orientation skills quips that she will be leading all of us out of burning buildings and planes when the lights go out. My deaf friends avoid the stress of noise pollution and the exhaustion of talking over the incessant din in fashionable bars in which social and professional life takes place now. Another friend, who is a small person, remarks that he consumes fewer resources and fits better into airplane spaces than big guys good at fighting and football. Some people with autism have a capacity to focus that boosts creativity. Expertise at composing with my voice instead of clunky keyboards puts me ahead in new communication technology.

The bright line between the healthy and the diseased, those who "have" a disease and those that don't, grows dimmer every day. Each of us carries within us many "orphan diseases"—that faintly Dickensian phrase that typically severs the connection between people like me and the human family of ordinary people. All of us are anything but "orphans." Instead, we are all second or third cousins, inextricably linked through a chain of quickly vanishing ancestors and descendants. We are all patients-in-waiting, bound together on a wait list of inheritance hidden deep in the elegant whirls of that double helix in every one of our cells—silently paused in its inscrutable determination to shape our lives. All those clichés of connectedness are now encoded in our genes. The human community is quite literally the human family.

We disabled are no longer orphans. We are instead a sturdy tribe, blood kin, navigating a changing world, living well, bonding fast and passing it on.

My Life With Tourette Syndrome

SHANE FISTELL

W HEN I WAS 17, MY FATHER TOOK ME TO A JUVENILE TREATMENT clinic to see if doctors could figure out what was wrong with me. I entered a room. I sat on a chair. I waited for a long while. There was a video camera trained on me. Then I heard voices, the voices of doctors behind a two-way mirror. It was like being in a police interrogation room in the movies.

A voice boomed: "So Shane, why do you think you're acting this way? Do you know what you're doing?"

I didn't know what to say. What were the right answers?

I was born with a neurological disorder that causes involuntary movements, vocalizations and tics—sometimes mild, sometimes wildly disruptive: Tourette syndrome. Since my youth, I've often been stopped in public by the police and questioned because of my symptoms.

Questioned: That sums it up in a single word. My whole life has been questioned. I'm 56 now. I've often led a life of self-imposed house arrest. Two months here, three months there. Summer gone, winter over. How many years have I wasted?

If people know of Tourette's, they will often say: "Oh, that's that swearing disease!" A woman once said to me: "At least you don't swear! You would've been worse off!"

Compulsive swearing is called coprolalia. Each person with Tourette's is different, and only some swear compulsively. I don't; but for most of my life I have had to put up with people swearing and cursing at me because of my symptoms. A few years ago a man argued: "There's no way you have Tourette's! If you don't swear you don't have it! Period. And I know you don't have it because I've seen it on TV!"

The average person doesn't know where in the body his kidneys are located. They couldn't tell you exactly how a baby is born. But they can decide if you do or do not have Tourette syndrome.

I am not aware of any other medical condition that provokes such wrath. The minimum social standard is one that I often don't meet. "You think you can say and do anything you want to just because you got Tourette's!" they accuse. Or: "He's always got this Tourette's thing, that's what makes him act that way."

"He just can't help it" is another form of counterfeit sympathy.

Do these same people truly think that I want to face being ridiculed, embarrassed and being shunned and ignored, not being believed, having little or no credibility, being barred, threatened, ostracized, rejected, isolated, rebuked and laughed at, even assaulted—even as they acknowledge that I *have* Tourette's?

I've been interrogated by just about everybody—by doctors, by the police and by the public. I have been examined, poked, prodded till I farted. Would you call me paranoid if I said that there are people who think I'm an alien from another planet?

Unlike most other medical conditions or disabilities, Tourette's is suspect, is subject to scrutiny. Motives are frequently attached. People ascribe or attribute my symptoms to a person who's out of control or to criminality.

It must be said that I can hurt myself, too. Sometimes, at day's end, my body is worn out from the punishing tics. At other extreme times I have injured myself slamming into walls and doors.

Sleep is merciful on my body, but I often wake up in the middle of the night. The twitches and tics can change minute to minute, hour to hour and day to day. Tourette's obeys its own schedule, obeys its own course and obeys its own relentless drive.

People's reactions toward me can be just as unpredictable; some think that alternative reasons for my tics and twitches must exist. I had an acquaintance who was a religious nut. He once said, "I believe you're possessed."

I said, "Yeah, well, I believe I'm dispossessed." I had no friends and no money. "I want to exorcise you. I have some holy water," he said.

I knew exactly what he meant and I knew what he wanted to do. He pulled out a white plastic Kentucky Fried Chicken figurine piggy bank of Colonel Sanders. It was filled with holy water— blessed Toronto tap water. Suddenly he threw the water across my body. He hosed me over in a sign of the cross pattern.

The water was icy cold. I was soaked. My shriek of protest was evidence enough for him of my demonic possession.

"I've done it!" he cried. "Devil out. Be gone!"

I twitched and jerked. "If only," I said.

Years ago I began to question whether prescription drugs I took to suppress my symptoms were for my benefit alone. I realized the drugs were in large part meant to benefit the public and to suppress their negative reaction toward my symptoms. It was a chemical exorcism.

Just swallow the pill.

First I tried an antipsychotic (often prescribed then for Tourette's, even though it's not a psychotic disorder). It left me drooling and nearly comatose; I had to sleep 16 to 18 hours a day. Then I tried another drug, which dropped my blood pressure to dangerously low levels. I made the choice then to sacrifice social acceptability for the freedom to be myself.

No two people with Tourette's are alike. Modern drugs do help some people with Tourette's. But I don't take any medications anymore.

There is no single drug designed specifically for Tourette's. Actually, I am sometimes accused of using drugs of a different type, of being a drug addict. When someone says, "Are you on drugs?" that is not a real question. It is not sympathetic. It is an accusation.

Drug dealers often approach me. They see my behaviors, and

are sure that I'm on some kind of street drugs. "What do you need? Want some crack? Meth? You sure? What are you on? What?"

I've never used drugs to hide from myself, nor to hide from people. I will not use drugs to win acceptance and approval. However, I admire and laud the dedicated research efforts on our behalf, even though designing a drug for Tourette's would not make much profit. I wish they could design a drug that could be given to other people so they don't see Tourette's.

With all the sacrifices and all the losses, there are also upsides to my Tourette's. I vibrate with almost inexhaustible energy and life and vitality. I have unusually excellent eyesight, and few things escape my attention. I have a heightened sense of hearing and smell. I have the heart of an athlete. My symptoms go up and down and everywhere, but my intelligence maintains itself. Sure I have Tourette's, but I think I may have swindled God in the exchange.

Day to day, if I do have a complaint it's that I have muscle fatigue, pain and exhaustion sometimes from my tics. Also: I have a heightened libido, but I don't have a woman.

A recent news report stated that Charles Manson, age 73, married a 23-year-old woman. The wedding ceremony took place inside the prison. I naïvely, vainly thought this was cause for celebration. If an elderly mass murderer serving a life sentence can get married, then maybe I'll meet a woman and get married, too. I doubt it. Most women stand me up and turn me down.

As I get older, the hardest challenge remains life itself. Thousands of people have tested social boundaries on me, yet if I complain or resist I can be accused of anything from being the aggressor to playing the victim. I am expected to apologize.

Sorry, *sorry* and *sorry*. I will not have a life of having to apologize.

People rarely apologize to me. And I am not allowed to be shocked when people mimic me freely with what they think is complete anonymity and immunity. They want to encourage people to ridicule me without having it heaped onto them. They attempt to usurp my Tourette's as though they can wear it like a monkey suit.

A few years ago, I was the subject of a documentary. It premiered at a film festival. After the screening, I walked out into the lobby. A young man approached me. He said, "I know you're faking it because I am an actor." And then he acted like someone acting like they have Tourette's.

What was I supposed to do? Laugh? Clap?

Often mimicry like this is trapped in my memory in an endless loop, and in this way my Tourette's becomes their Tourette's.

I said, "Actually, the only time I am faking is when I pretend I don't have Tourette's."

The Everyday Anxiety of
the Stutterer

JOSEPH P. CARTER

THERE AT THE REGISTER, THE FRUSTRATION WELLED UP IN ME. AGAIN. And it was only morning. The cashier waited for my response, but my mouth hinged open, lock-jawed and gaping for the whole world to see. And as usual, nothing came out.

I stutter.

Some stutterers repeat words or syllables. Mine is a complete block that lasts anywhere from a second to what seems like eternity. (Really, though, there isn't much of a difference.) Sometimes noticeable facial tics accompany these blocks. In moments of fluency, I make solid eye contact; but when I stutter, none whatsoever.

Many people are understandably unsure what to say in these situations. There is the furtive look-around and the uneasy chuckle, followed by "Did you forget your name?" or "Are you just nervous?" Others patiently wait, which for some reason makes it more frustrating to me. Once I *tell* them about my stuttering, the confusion is resolved. Some even note the irony.

One of the greatest difficulties stutterers face is introducing themselves. Casual introductions are so ingrained in our everyday experience that it seems silly even to point them out. They are, by their very nature, mundane. For the stutterer like myself, however, they are anything but that. "Hi, I'm Joey." I hardly get to say this. Something so hackneyed is, for me, a palpable struggle.

There are the little things, too. When the gas station clerk asks, "Credit or debit?" you probably take it in stride. I don't. I wince. To avoid the struggle, I simply smile at a stranger who opens a door for me. Saying "Thank you"—quickly and easily, exactly as I imagine saying it—feels entirely beyond my powers.

My everyday life is filled with such conspicuousness.

Conspicuous the word is from the Latin *conspicere*, or "all eyes here." The early 20th-century German philosopher Martin Heidegger said that conspicuousness is the peculiar moment that ruptures the fundamental fabric of human experience—the everyday.

It is this quality of "everydayness," the banal flow of day-to-day life, that pervades all of human existence. We are so absorbed in it that it is forgotten. It is the elusive backdrop of consciousness, the home in which we dwell. It's the familiar fabric that weaves together every expectation, interpretation and interaction we have as human beings, everything from casual introductions to theoretical speculations. That it is so readily forgotten is, in fact, part of the nature of everydayness. So, when we notice it, it's rather peculiar—conspicuous.

But, then how do we come to notice it at all? And when we do, what exactly is the value of bringing it to our attention?

According to Heidegger, the everyday shows itself when its familiarity troubles us. Sigmund Freud called it das Unheimliche, "the uncanny" or literally "the unhomely." It is that peculiar moment when the very familiarity of our everyday world is itself unfamiliar—uncanny. When our cars break down, planes and commuter trains are delayed, or the tires on our bicycles unexpectedly pop—it is at points like these that we recognize they are valuable precisely to the extent that we, for the most part, can take their functioning for granted. They are essential tools for our daily routines. When these things break down, we get to see (perhaps for the first time) how they really worked, and more important, why we value them so much.

Communication, particularly the spoken word, is not altogether different from the train that almost always arrives on time. Speech is a basic feature of human experience. We are so often at home with our ways of speaking. Yet, like the broken-down car or delayed commuter train, stuttering illuminates this everyday world of speech in ways that expose not only its importance, but also the particular way that it works.

For starters, it reveals an important distinction between language and speech. Language concerns propositional content—the meanings of words (semantics), the rules by which words form sentences (syntax), and how accurately what we say corresponds to the world (truth and falsity). But, speech conveys so much more than this. We speak in order to communicate not merely our words, but our feelings, intentions, and ultimately, our selves.

Think about how you speak and how others speak to you. Is it only your language—words and syntax—that matters? Or rather that what you say is meaningful all the way down to the texture of your voice? There is a reason we sometimes apologize for *how* we say something rather than what we say—the timing, cadence and tonality of our speech can make all the difference in the world.

And yet, as humans, we are often unaware of the everydayness of speech. As a stutterer, I'm made aware of it all the more. Every day.

No matter the situation, the familiarity of speech appears to me in anxiety-filled moments that I've come to predict with almost scientific precision. Speech is such an uncanny phenomenon for me. I'm never at home with my stuttering; I feel ashamed on a daily basis. I am conspicuous.

But conspicuousness need not always be troublesome. This is something Heidegger misses. There are times when it allows me to experience the generosity of others (something we also tend to take for granted).

Remember the cashier? Several years ago, I ventured to Georgia Square Mall in Athens, Ga., to get fitted for a tux. My friend's wedding was coming up fast. Early in the morning, I grudgingly drove there. As I approached the counter, the young woman attending the register kindly asked how she could help me. I struggled to speak. Still groggy from the early morning, my stuttering was quite obvious. I made a writing motion with my right hand over my left palm in order to ask for pen and paper. Instead of the usual, predictable responses, she began to communicate with me in sign language. She assumed I was deaf.

She was very skilled—*fluent*. It made me smile. In a moment of my own fluency, I told her that I stutter. She blushed and apologized for her mistake. But, there was no need for an apology. Because, in an instant, she recognized my trouble, my everydayness, and made sure to help me as best she knew how. The conspicuousness of my stuttering allowed another person to see my struggle and to meet me with kindness in return.

For the remainder of my time at the tuxedo shop, I did not stutter. In fact, I was able to tell her my name without any trouble.

Everyone comes face to face with the everyday world through some struggle or another. We must confront our everydayness through these troubling lenses because it forces us to recognize things that should never be mundane and ordinary. Taking notice of what is mundane *via* our own struggles has the remarkable power to instruct and enjoin us to confront injustices, to assess our own privilege, and to *change* our everyday behaviors.

Just look at our current sociopolitical climate. The fact that racism, misogyny, bigotry, discrimination, class inequity and sexual violence are still prevalent today is rooted in how those with privilege—those of us who do not have to face systemic oppression, myself included—rarely, if ever, encounter these injustices every single day. The oppressed are routinely forgotten and accepted as part of the human experience. They recede into the background. They are not troubling to us. Oppression, thereby, remains inconspicuous. Everyday. And this is dangerous.

How to Really See a
Blind Person

BRAD SNYDER

I TELL MY STORY A LOT. I TELL THE STORY OF HOW I WASN'T ALWAYS BLIND. I tell the story of how I lost my vision while serving in Afghanistan, by stepping on an I.E.D. I tell the story of how I put my own injury into perspective by considering the greater sacrifice of my fallen comrades, and how I owed it to them to make the most of my escape from death.

I tell the story of how I did that by winning a gold medal in swimming at the Paralympics on the first anniversary of the loss of my vision. And after I tell it, people often thank me. They tell me that it's an incredible story, and that I'm a good storyteller. They tell me how inspiring it is to see how I've overcome my blindness.

But that's not my whole story.

It's part of it, I suppose—in many ways, I *have* overcome my blindness. Five years after losing my sight, I have a rewarding job teaching leadership at the Naval Academy, a lovely house on a creek in historic Annapolis, Md., a loving family and a number of truly deep friendships. My quality of life is very high. Day to day, week to week, I don't find that my blindness is an obstacle.

What I haven't been able to overcome is how others perceive me and treat me differently now because of my blindness, or how I so often feel as if I'm on the outside listening in on the lives of others.

I hear people talk about how beautiful the sunrise is, but I no longer see it. I hear them talk about "Game of Thrones," but cannot watch it because HBO doesn't currently have descriptive audio for its shows. I can no longer share these very common experiences.

One thing I do often now is public talks about learning to navigate my new life without vision. But it's a one-way conversation. Afterward, I go to the airport where I'm reminded how hard it is to physically navigate a world not set up for people without vision. It's a pain to find assistance at the counter. It's a pain to get through security, which can't seem to distinguish dog food from explosives. It's a pain to get the airlines to move my seat to the bulkhead so there's room for my guide dog. Don't get me started on what a pain it is to find the bathroom for either of us.

I feel the looks of my fellow passengers, wondering what my story is, but too afraid to ask for fear of saying the wrong thing and offending me. I feel helpless, stared at like some sort of freak.

In my former life as an explosive ordnance disposal officer, I traveled through airports all over the world, from Baltimore to Prague to Baghdad to Kandahar and back, quickly, easily and anonymously. But traveling as I do now, with a cane and a guide dog, is anything but anonymous. At times, it has beaten me down.

At home, the inability to join my friends in their chatter about "Game of Thrones" or memes on Instagram has caused me to pull back. I decline invitations out to avoid the same alienating experience I've had a thousand times before. Whether I'm at a crowded bar, restaurant, sports event or concert, I'll be a spectacle, isolated by my inability to join the conversations of those around me.

No, thanks. I'll just stay home, in the quiet, where I know exactly where the bathroom is. I'll stay there until I have to hit the road again to tell my story of how I overcame blindness.

The irony used to make me chuckle.

A few years ago, after another frustrating trip through the airport, I settled into my seat bound for Dallas and did my best to disappear.

"That's an awfully nice watch you have there! I've never seen anything quite like it!" my neighbor said as she fastened her seatbelt.

A smile spread across my face. I love talking about my watch. It's a tactile timepiece that replaces traditional hour and minute hands with magnetic, rotating ball bearings so that blind folks like myself can literally tell the time through touch. It's superbly designed and very sharp-looking, so it appeals to those with vision too.

The timepiece—the Bradley by Eone—is actually named after me. It is accessible to people with or without disabilities. (I am a friend of the company's founder, Hyungsoo Kim, and receive a small percentage on sales of the watch.) I love explaining how the watch embodies the principles of inclusive design, which I am passionate about.

The conversation with my neighbor went on, and I explained how I lost my vision. I talked about how I had been able to adapt, how I try to maintain perspective and how I felt as though I had overcome my blindness.

Then my neighbor shared her own fights. She had lost her husband a few years ago, and during her grief had gained weight. She had been struggling with her weight ever since, and it had begun to interfere with her quality of life. I told her how sometimes I felt isolated by my disability, and she relayed that she felt constrained by her weight. I shared how I sometimes feel that I'm an outsider, and she echoed the same.

For the first time in a while, I didn't feel like a spectacle or an outcast. I felt like a friend, and an important part of someone else's journey. I felt valued, needed and involved, and all it took was a conversation. I realized that I'm not alone in being alone.

Sometimes people ask me what I want others to know about being blind. I want others to feel more comfortable having conversations with people whose experiences are different from their own. My watch has been a natural opener, and once that conversation starts, we usually discuss topics far beyond timepieces and disabilities. Through talking, we find humanity.

It seems like we could all use a little more humanity right now. I know it's tough for many to have conversations with people so different from themselves, to risk feeling uncomfortable or giving offense, to find common ground, to listen to another's struggles, to share your own struggles in return. But you might be surprised what you get out of it—and what you realize you've given in return.

How do we do it? It all starts with a conversation. What's your story?

The Importance of Facial Equality

ARIEL HENLEY

I HAVE NEVER SEEN SOMEONE WHO LOOKED LIKE ME ON A MAINSTREAM television show. I have never seen someone who looked like me, playing anything but a villain in movies, or in an ad or on a billboard. I am invisible. That is, until I walk down the street. That is, until strangers stare just a little too long and rudely whisper, "Look at her eyes."

As a child, I was often asked why my eyes were shaped the way they were, so crooked and far apart.

"I don't know," I would shrug. "I just came that way!" Sometimes this question bothered me, because I didn't understand why everyone felt the need to ask it. Most of the time, I just didn't know how to respond.

I was born with a craniofacial disease—Crouzon syndrome, a condition where the bones in the head do not grow. A condition that required too many surgeries and procedures to count, so I grew accustomed to being cut open, pulled apart, and put back together. Though I quickly learned that once something is taken apart, it's never quite the same.

The first time someone told me I was ugly, I was in the seventh grade. I didn't even realize I was "different" until I reached middle school. I always just assumed I was normal—I *felt* normal, but I quickly learned I did not look it.

"Does it hurt to be *disfigured*?" bullies would sometimes ask me.

"Does it hurt to be an idiot?" I would sometimes respond.

If you Google the word "disfigured," you get a definition "spoil the attractiveness of," derived from the Latin word *fingere*, meaning "to shape." Many consider the word to be offensive; others do not. I was born with a facial disfigurement, and not only do I *not* find the term offensive, but I also do not believe myself to be unattractive.

I did a lot of growing up during my time at the local children's hospital, where the bones of my head and face were routinely broken and restructured, rectifying the premature fusion of my skull. After surgeries, during my extended stays in the intensive care unit, I would tell myself that pain was not real. That it was imaginary and only in my mind. If I concentrated hard enough on the throbbing pain throughout my body, I could convince myself, if only for a moment, that I was numb. I would lie there, unable to sit up, my eyes swollen shut. Nurses and visitors bestowed words of comfort upon me, trying to ease my terror, but over time, I grew used to it. What was once horrific became normal.

Even with the physically traumatic surgeries I was required to undergo, the physical aspect of my condition was nothing compared with the emotional toll of living with an appearance-altering condition. The everyday stares, comments, and subhuman treatment acted as a constant reminder of my painful medical history and my perceived shortcomings.

I lived much of my early life in survival mode. The priority was to keep me alive.

Because salvaging my physical health was so crucial, the emotional aspect of living with a facial disfigurement was overlooked by health professionals. While my mother and father did their best to offer support, there was only so much they could do. I tried therapy, but therapists always seemed to ask the wrong questions and never seemed to understand what it was like to have my physical appearance change drastically time and time again. "It's like in 'Freaky Friday,'" I would tell them. "Except I never get my body back. I never get my face back." Despite their best efforts, they simply could not relate.

To make matters more challenging, I never had anyone who had been through the same experiences to turn to for advice and support. I would search the internet for others like me, trying to find personal stories and tips and advice for how to get through it, but was never able to find anything. I felt alone. To get through it, I told myself I would grow up to be the stereotypical definition of beautiful. With each surgery I had, I assured myself I was getting one step closer to being able to walk down the street in peace. People would no longer stare at me in confusion and disgust, wondering why I looked the way I did. Instead, they would admire my beauty. I would finally be happy. Nobody told me happiness was an inside job.

The Americans With Disabilities Act classifies facial disfigurement as a form of disability, recognizing the fact that individuals with facial disfigurements encounter discrimination and prejudice because of their appearance. I face discrimination and prejudice when I apply for jobs, when I'm on a date, when I walk down the street. The judgment is everywhere. Still, I refuse to live my life in seclusion, because other individuals are uncomfortable with my existence.

People with Crouzon syndrome and other conditions that result in facial disfigurements are not represented in mainstream media. How can individuals with disfigurements and physical differences be expected to accept ourselves and love our differences, when we aren't even *worthy* of mainstream inclusion? Not only that, but there are people who would be angered if such inclusion were to exist. How are individuals with facial disfigurements supposed to be seen as equal when we still face discrimination in every area of our lives every single day?

There is no standard when it comes to the language and the representation surrounding facial disfigurements. I often use the word "disfigurement" in my work, because I find it packs more of a punch. It feels more powerful. Harsh, even. Terms like "facial difference" and "facial diversity" never feel adequate in describing my experiences.

While it may imply that there is an existing standard in terms of physical appearance that individuals with conditions like Crouzon syndrome do not measure up to, I choose the word "disfigurement" because of the power it holds. I'm viewed as having a disfigurement, not just a difference. I believe the intensity of the term "disfigurement" allows individuals to become more aware of their own prejudice and more mindful of how they treat others.

Through this and other methods, I am working toward creating a world where those who are not disfigured recognize those who are as equals, where a person with Crouzon syndrome is given a role in a popular television show or is hired to appear in an ad or fashion campaign. In that world, I'd be able to go about my business or show up to a job interview without having my entire being called into question by strangers, and others with facial disfigurements would be truly viewed as a valuable addition to society. Because we are.

Finding Refuge With
the Skin I'm In

ANNE KAIER

THE CHECKOUT LADY'S PANIC SURGED AS SHE HELD THE COINS SIX inches above my hand and dropped them into my palm. They clanged until I made a fist. She ran her fingernails through her hair.

"What's wrong with you?" she asked, her voice rising to a higher pitch. I slid the money into a jeans pocket and stroked my thigh to calm down.

"Just dry skin," I murmured. That wasn't true. I have lamellar ichthyosis, a genetic disorder which manifests itself in scales not just on my face, arms, hands—which she could see—but over my whole body. My skin is perpetually red and itchy. I can't sweat well, so I'm careful not to get overheated, and I can't walk far in strong sun. I naturally seek the shade. My skin isn't painful, but much of the time, the entire surface of my body feels tight. My eyelids are pulled down by this tightness, too, so I often shield my face with a hat. Standing in the checkout line, I jammed the lovely straw boater I'd gotten in England down to blunt my face. *Damn it*, I thought, *get me out of h*ere.

I knew I could smile and tell her my condition was not contagious, but instead I hurried home through narrow city streets, slammed my heavy front door, and headed straight into the tiny walled garden in the back.

The garden is my refuge. It's the reason I bought this house. Even a small leafy space is unusual among Philadelphia row homes and

I craved a private place with fresh air and shaded light. I water my three trees in hot spells and nurture cool white moonflowers. The unseeing trees and plants comfort me. Pacing the bricks, I fought the instinct to go into the house and hide. *I can't spend my entire life in bed*, I told myself, brushing Japanese maple leaves against my cheek to soothe my skin and my spirit. Hiding was a cop-out—not the mature thing to do.

I don't usually hide. I live in Center City Philadelphia where I see—and am seen—by people on the street all the time. I teach at a local university. I go out to dinner with my friends. But the cashier's reaction shook me. I told myself she was new to that supermarket, didn't know me, hadn't been the recipient of my considerable charm. Still her words stung. Among my pots of fragrant herbs, I stripped a thyme frond, crushed the petals and inhaled their fragrance. I felt an overwhelming need to chuck my afternoon class, avoid my merry students' faces, and burrow under my flowered quilt.

I settled in to the wrought-iron chair next to the garden wall and recalled a humid Philly summer day in 1953, when I was 7 and my mother took a flock of kids—me, my brother, and two of our two young cousins—to swim in a suburban pond turned swimming club called Martin's Dam. Nonmembers like us paid a small fee at the admissions gate beyond which the spring-fed "swimming hole" rippled under hanging maples. Carrying our towels, we kids scampered after my mom who strode up to the gate to pay for us. When I got near the gatekeeper, she fixed her gaze on my abnormally red face and the shards of skin scattered like salt on my arms and legs. I lowered my eyes, tugging shame and surprise and fear into tight cords in my chest. "What's going on here?" the woman asked.

"Nothing that'll hurt you," my mother shot back. "Just dry skin." The gatekeeper let us in. I ducked past her and ran nearer to the pond, pretending nothing had happened. My mother did, too. I slithered into the cool green water up to my neck. When we left I draped my towel around my shoulders and scurried past the woman at the gate who had wondered if my scales would grow on her if I brushed her thigh.

That was more than 60 years ago, but I can still inspire fear in ordinary strangers, people who glance at me at the movies or on a city sidewalk. I tense up every time I stride past the iron railings through the park across from my house. I feel my jaw tighten at the sight of all those people. Will the guy in shorts ambling along with his groceries stare at my crimson face? Will the red-haired boy chalking an airplane on the bricks look up as I pass him by in flip-flops? In truth, most of these people are simply more interested in their own affairs than in me. But the starers have entered my inner eye. Whether they stare at me or not almost doesn't matter.

Experts give high-minded advice about how to respond. When someone stares at me, I am to educate them. "You must be wondering about my appearance. It's not contagious. I just have problem skin. It's called ichthyosis and I was born with it." I'm supposed to tell them what's going on: Ichthyosis comes from a recessive gene, like blue eyes. All very nice and instructive. But I can't do this day after day, with starer after starer as I walk through the park on my way to meet a friend in the local cafe or past throngs of undergraduates on my way to teach Shakespeare.

No number of reassuring explanations can protect me from the underlying dread of infection that lurks beneath some of these stares. What's it like to be the object of such fear? It forces me to dig for deep waters of self-love. It also makes me angry. Not long ago I leaned back from my screen when I came across a comment on the website of this paper from a reader about an article showcasing beautiful photos of people with albinism, port wine stains or Down syndrome. "Our perception of human beauty (and ugliness and deformity) evolved to encourage the selection of genetically fit mates," he wrote, "and to reduce the spread of contagious disease."

I tried to shake off this iteration of a debunked "evolutionary" basis for shunning. Then I noticed that nearly 100 people had "recommended" it with a thumbs up. I spun my chair around and kicked aside a basket of laundry, knowing these comments would linger like a fungus in my mind. This person might be surprised to know that my parents were both handsome, and that the kind of revulsion he was spreading can impel otherwise perfectly decent citizens to isolate anyone who looks radically different.

Even a person who scares some people has to make her way in the world. It's become fashionable to tell a disability story in a hopeful arc, where the heroine may have moments of discouragement or fear, but comes out into full life at the end—into mainstream schools, love and romance, full participation in the social world. Although I have done and had all of these, I still, now and then, allow myself to hide; I refuse, for a while, to encounter the world.

That day after the cashier stared at me, I did go to teach my undergraduates. I could never bail on my students. But back home in the late afternoon, I dropped plans to go out to a noisy restaurant with a bunch of friends. Instead, I took a book into my secret garden, read for a few minutes, and then bent to smell the purple hyacinths beneath my maple tree. Rising, I turned my face to the quiet clouds moving along the sky. I need these hours of retreat. And I claim them, not just as necessary to top up my courage to go back out into the world, but for their own still sweetness, their soft and leafy balm.

What It Means to Heal

CYNDI JONES

"IF YOU HAD FAITH, YOU WOULD BE HEALED."

The words came from a stranger who came up to me at the mall, where I was going about my business on the scooter I use for mobility. He then asked to lay hands on me and pray.

I was shocked the first time this happened. Not anymore. Such encounters occur regularly to me and other disabled people. I want to tell these would-be healers: "I have faith. *Do you* need prayers?" Instead, I say: "I'm fine. Thanks."

I can't remember a time when I wanted healing because of my disability. But I can quickly recall times when I wished our society were healed of its attitudes toward disability. If society were healed, people with disabilities could more easily find jobs and housing. We could go places on the subway and when we arrived, we could enter through the front door. We would be expected to participate in typical social and work activities. We could live our own lives making good or bad choices, just like everybody else.

Little do these strangers know—I do have faith, and the wounds that they see actually bear witness to a miracle. If they only understood that my scars are reminders of prayers answered.

There's a story in the New Testament, in the Gospel of Mark, about Jairus, one of the leaders of the synagogue who came to Jesus and fell at his feet and begged him repeatedly: "My little daughter is at the point of death. Come and lay your hands on her, so that she may be made well, and live."

When I was 2 years old I became very sick and was unable to

breathe on my own. My father, like Jairus, pleaded with God to save the life of his daughter. My throat was cut open so that a machine could breathe for me. *How fragile life is, supported by nothing but thin air.*

For months an iron lung supported every breath I took, and when the electricity in the hospital failed, Dad would come to the hospital at all hours of the night to hand crank the machine keeping me alive. Dad never spoke about this. He had a humble, quiet faith, and I am the beneficiary of his pleading.

Many of the stories of healing in the New Testament actually have nothing to do with the faith of the person who is healed and everything to do with those who have a relationship with that person. It was the faith of Jairus that was enough for Jesus to heal his daughter. It was the tenacity of the boundary-breaking Canaanite mother that led Jesus to heal her daughter. It was the sheer boldness of the four friends who cut a hole in the roof to set their paralyzed friend in front of Jesus to be healed. And sometimes it was Jesus wanting to make a point that was the catalyst for healing. In all these stories and more, the person who received healing usually had no say in the matter, no agency.

In the New Testament, Jesus would often say before bringing about a physical healing, "Your sins are forgiven." The first and most important healing was invisible.

This happened to Bartimaeus, who was blind and sitting by the roadside begging. When he called out to Jesus, those around him told him to shut up and sit down, stay in your place. But Jesus called him to come near.

When he approached, Jesus asked him, "What do you want me to do for you?" Jesus did not assume that Bartimaeus's lack of physical vision was the most important thing that needed to be restored.

In fact, the first healing for Bartimaeus was regaining his agency, being asked what *he* wanted and answering for himself. His dignity was restored, and then his vision.

People often pray for healing without recognizing that what

needs to be healed is the community around them, including themselves. But this sacred, mystical, invisible healing can happen in our communities. It is not brought about by restoring the ability to see or walk or sing on key, but being welcoming, accepting and embracing all others into belonging.

A few years ago a member of the church congregation brought Beth, a friend with an intellectual disability, to church. Beth was new to church and was somewhat disruptive during the service. This community was accustomed to all sorts of interruptions, "free roaming" toddlers and people wandering in with urgent needs. When Beth started coming, people were drawn to her, and a small group quickly formed to accompany her. Gradually she learned the rhythms of the church and the people who loved her. The community missed her when she didn't come. Beth had become part of the fabric of the community.

When those around you understand that you, exactly as you are, are essential to all of creation in a way that we cannot understand, that without you creation would be incomplete—that is healing.

Healing moves you through the turmoil, the regular assault on your being, to move past that which is preventing you from being all that you are meant to be, to knowing that you belong here. Your very existence is good and necessary.

The person who approached me at the mall was seeing only the person in front of him. He was not seeing the bigger picture. Although it may not be obvious, my disability is a gift to a community and a vehicle to reach out to others who are struggling. Over the years my personal understanding of disability has opened a place, a path through their struggles, for many people by providing a new perspective.

Perhaps our prayers for healing might be not for miraculous "cures" for individuals but for society at large to be more welcoming, inclusive and hospitable to everyone. Then instead of focusing on others' visible scars, we see all people as they are, with everything that has brought them to be present with us in this moment.

III

WORKING

I Use a Wheelchair. And Yes, I'm Your Doctor.

CHERI A. BLAUWET

WHEN I WAS IN THE THIRD YEAR OF MY MEDICAL RESIDENCY, I WAS asked to evaluate a new state-of-the-art, fully accessible exam table that would be used in doctors' offices to better provide care for patients with mobility-related disabilities. The table could go as low as 18 inches off the ground to enable easier transfers for wheelchair users and had extra rails and grips to provide support for patients with impaired balance.

I was to assess this equipment as a "user expert." Although the table was designed to accommodate patients with disabilities, I rolled up to it to evaluate it from the perspective of a physician. "Do you want my opinion as a patient, or as a doctor?" I asked the surprised representatives from the medical equipment company.

I have been a wheelchair user since early childhood, when I sustained a spinal cord injury in a farming accident. I am now a practicing physician in the field of rehabilitation and sports medicine.

In my busy outpatient clinical practice, I witness the spectrum of patients' reactions when they find out that their doctor is, herself, disabled. Typically those first few seconds after entering an exam room—before the patient's guard goes up—are the most informative.

I find that these reactions are somewhat generational. Younger patients, having grown up amid a growing awareness of disability in society, typically do not react at all. They have clearly encountered empowered people with disabilities working in various professional roles. Older patients often seem confused, curious or, in rare circumstances, dismayed.

Several months ago, I wheeled into the room of an elderly woman. She looked at me, placed her hand on mine and, with a kind look asked, "Are you an invalid?" More recently, a jovial older man exclaimed, "You've got to be kidding me!" A few times, patients will hesitate to tell me their concerns, indicating "Well, doc, I feel bad complaining about this to you, when clearly your problems are bigger than mine."

Several years ago, while in my residency, I was in line at our hospital cafeteria. Although my badge reading "Dr. Blauwet" and stethoscope were clearly visible, a man next to me in line said: "You look like you are doing pretty well. When are you going to be discharged?" Clearly, my wheelchair was the only thing he saw. Moreover, he equated my wheelchair with illness, rather than empowerment.

Over the years, I've thought a lot about situations like these, and I do not believe they come so much from direct prejudice as from people's lack of experience with doctors who are also wheelchair users. A recent study revealed that less than 3 percent of medical school trainees are people with disabilities, and of these, only a small proportion are individuals with mobility impairment. How can we expect our patients or colleagues to know about the perspectives and needs of physicians with disabilities when we remain invisible to them?

The reason for this underrepresentation is complicated. Most physicians with mobility disabilities will tell you that the problem is not that we lack the ability to do our job competently. As with many other educated, skilled professionals, we know how to choose a path that suits our talents and abilities. Reasonable accommodations, such as the use of standing wheelchairs in the operating room, give us the access we need to do our work. The larger barrier to entry for prospective doctors with disabilities, however, is bias, both overt and hidden.

A colleague who is quadriplegic recounted a medical school admissions officer telling him, "I'm afraid that you will not meet the technical standards for admission." Although steeped in bias and probably illegal, this response was at least more direct than the more common form of discrimination where otherwise strong applicants with disabilities simply do not receive an interview or a call back. As our peers are accepted into prestigious schools and academic positions, we sit on the sidelines, left to question whether the fault lies with us or the system. Many give up their aspirations of a career in medicine altogether, electing to pursue work more "traditionally suited" for people with disabilities. Others lose sleep, questioning whether it was the right decision to disclose their disability in the application materials.

Anyone can enter, at any time, the minority group of people with disabilities. The most common cause of new, adult-onset disability is—simply put—aging. Physicians are often reluctant to disclose new-onset or progressive disability (like loss of hearing or vision, or reduced mobility) because of the fear of being stigmatized; medicine, after all, is still dominated by the prototype of physical prowess.

Dr. Lisa Iezzoni, a professor of medicine at Harvard Medical School, has been an important mentor to me for many years. She recounted her experience as a medical student at Harvard in the early 1980s, a decade before the passage of the Americans With Disabilities Act. In her first year at the medical school, after experiencing some physical and sensory symptoms, she was given a diagnosis of multiple sclerosis. Late in her third year, after a fall, she started using a cane, but her aspirations to pursue an internal medicine residency remained, despite the overt discouragement she received. At a student-faculty dinner, an influential professor told her: "There are too many doctors in the country right now for us to worry about training a handicapped physician. If that means someone gets left by the wayside, that's too bad."

The medical school refused to write a letter of recommendation for her residency application, so she could not pursue the training required for clinical practice. She pursued health policy research instead and became the first female professor of medicine at the Beth Israel Deaconess Medical Center and now directs the Mongan Institute Health Policy Center at Massachusetts General Hospital. Despite having had an extraordinarily successful career, she sometimes wonders what could have been if she had been able to practice medicine.

My experience, more than two decades later, was vastly different. As an undergraduate at the University of Arizona, I became interested in applying to medical school. I investigated the application process and took coursework that would set me up for success. I studied, networked, did internships and engaged in various activities that would strengthen my application. Additionally, throughout this time, I nurtured my alter ego as an athlete, pursuing the sport of wheelchair racing, and ultimately represented the United States in three Paralympic Games.

In the fall of 2002, I applied to medical school, received interviews at several prestigious universities and was accepted to the Stanford University School of Medicine. Throughout this process, I never once feared that my disability would get in the way of success. I could focus on my academic performance rather than expending mental energy around concerns of hidden bias.

As a member of the "ADA generation," I was blissfully ignorant that my visible disability could, in fact, derail my success. I simply assumed that I would be evaluated on merit, like my peers. (I also realized that my athletic success perhaps made me seem more "able.") I now understand the privilege of that perspective. I cannot completely separate my disability identity from my professional role.

People with disabilities often express fear or dissatisfaction with our health care system because they face poor access and discriminatory attitudes. This must change. Perhaps having more doctors with disabilities is one solution. As with any underrepresented group in medicine, professional diversity should reflect our population's diversity. That simple change can bring awareness, empathy and a shared experience that ultimately makes all of us better.

Standing Up for What I Need

CAROL R. STEINBERG

OPPOSING COUNSEL AND I WERE AT SIDEBAR, TALKING TO THE JUDGE out of the jury's earshot. The judge's face loomed high above me as she sat behind the "bench"—a four-foot-high wooden desk atop a two-foot-high platform. I was in a wheelchair and had to stretch my neck to communicate with her. Opposing counsel, who stood directly in front of the judge, quite comfortably made eye contact with her as she spoke.

I was not new at this. It was 2013 and I had tried over 50 jury cases in the past three decades, winning quite a few substantial verdicts, but I felt that something was going on. To be effective in my profession, you have to be heard. That can be difficult when you can't stand up to project your voice. This judge was ruling repeatedly in favor of the lawyer she could see and hear best.

I was already an experienced trial lawyer by the time I learned I had multiple sclerosis in 1995, at age 41. MS is a condition in which an abnormal response of the body's immune system is directed against the central nervous system and attacks myelin, the coating of the nerve fibers, and the fibers themselves. When the myelin or nerve fibers are attacked and damaged, scar tissue, or sclerosis, is formed, which prevents the proper transmission of messages through the brain, spinal cord and optic nerves, producing a wide variety of symptoms. In my case, it has primarily affected the use of my legs.

Since I started trying cases from a wheelchair 12 years ago, my relationship to my profession has changed. When I lose a case, I sometimes feel unsure of the reason for the defeat. Was I not persuasive because I couldn't get my point across from a wheelchair, or would my argument have lost no matter where it came from? Was I not treated as well by the judge or opposing counsel because I was sitting, or did I just not adequately articulate my point?

I don't want to believe that I'm being discriminated against because of my disability. Believing that not only requires advocacy for myself when I should be advocating for my clients, but also calls my ability to do what I love into question.

The first time I asked a judge to accommodate me was many years before when I was trying a prisoners' rights case and still walking on weak legs. That judge agreed before the jury came in that I could violate protocol and remain seated when I addressed her and them during the trial.

But when she later told the jury that I had difficulty standing because of a health condition, I was embarrassed. After that, I tried not to draw attention to my needs in the courtroom. That prevented me from asking this judge to come down from the bench so that I could communicate with her face to face.

I realize that I need to overcome this apprehension. For people trying to live a "normal" life with a disability, an aversion to "causing trouble" by asking for or demanding accommodation is understandable. But I know that resisting the reluctance to make waves is important—basic things like ramps, Braille materials, hearing assistance equipment or lowered counters can help people with disabilities live and work on or near par with others.

My wheelchair doesn't interfere with most pretrial tasks— preparing documents, having meetings, taking depositions. I have no trouble with many processes in court—speaking to a jury, questioning witnesses and talking to a judge from the middle of the courtroom, where everyone can hear me. The big challenge is the bench, particularly during sidebars, when the lawyers have to converse quietly with the judge at the side of her high bench.

Jury selection and conferences that are not for jury consumption take place there.

Before that day in 2013, I had overcome the obstacle of the bench in one of two ways: Sometimes, my tall law partner would try a case with me and help handle matters at sidebar. Other times, judges voluntarily came down and handled sidebar matters at the lower clerk's desk in front of the judge's bench. For whatever reason, this judge remained behind her high perch. And my own lack of confidence prevented me from asking her to make the accommodation.

The case that day concerned a 7-year-old boy who lost some of his vision when another child kicked a football into his eye during recess. I was arguing that the injury resulted from a lack of supervision on the part of school staff. The safety expert I hired was on the witness stand. The defense lawyer constantly interrupted her testimony, objecting and demanding to speak to the judge at sidebar. Once we were there, he would stand and argue that my questions or the expert's answers were not phrased properly. I would vigorously argue to the contrary from my seated position, feeling that I could hardly be heard.

This is not how it usually works. Ordinarily, the witness is able to testify and is then cross-examined by the other lawyer; I would have had no problem conducting the trial this way. But my opponent's tactic of continually interrupting and bringing us to sidebar, while I don't know if it was purposeful, was effective. We spent long periods with the judge agreeing with him and admonishing me from on high. The flow of my expert's testimony was disrupted. The jury looked confused as they were kept in the dark for extensive periods of time.

The impact on me was that my identity as a trial lawyer was shaken. As I stared at that wood in front of me, with the angry voice of my opponent and the obliging voice of the young judge above, I had one recurring thought: *Maybe it's time to do something else*. I felt I had no business trying a case in a wheelchair.

At the end of that day, opposing counsel unexpectedly approached me and offered to settle the case. The parents agreed. And I was glad to get their son a little money for his future.

I haven't tried a case since that day but will again. I'm always encouraged to see newer courthouses that have ramps at the judge's bench for lawyers like me. But if my next case isn't in one of those courthouses, I will ask the judge to come down. Those of us who need accommodation so that we can keep doing what we love must have the courage and self-respect to seek them, even if we would rather we didn't have to.

Where All Bodies Are Exquisite

RIVA LEHRER

IT's 2009, AND I'M IN PHILADELPHIA TO DELIVER A TALK AT A CONFERENCE. During a long break, I decide to visit the Mutter Museum. I teach anatomy, and the Mutter houses a collection of so-called medical curiosities. I examine the wall of skulls, the cases full of skeletons, and go downstairs, where preserved specimens wait for inspection.

And there I am confronted with a large case full of specimen jars. Each jar contains a late-term fetus, and all of the fetuses have the same disability: Their spinal column failed to fuse all the way around their spinal cord, leaving holes (called lesions) in their spine. Some extrude a bulging sac containing a section of the cord. These balloons make the fetuses appear as if they're about to explode. This condition is called spina bifida.

I stand in front of these tiny humans and try not to pass out. I have never seen what I looked like on the day I was born.

But this is essentially what my mother saw soon after I was born. I'm awe-struck that she didn't flinch, didn't institutionalize me, but kept me, fought for me, taught me how to fight. Still, I feel shock at the pure strangeness of my body, an old, old shame, and finally, sorrow. Not for myself; I feel it for my preserved kin, because their bodies were stopped in time. Historical artifacts marking a moment when medicine had nothing to offer.

Every human body is a marker in time. I was born in 1958, just as surgeons found a way to close the spina bifida lesion. At that time, the fatality rate hovered around 90 percent. It was medical practice to wait until a child reached 2 years old before doing any surgical intervention. A child that lived that long was considered strong enough to survive. But very few did. I was lucky to have had a surgeon who was trained in the newest techniques and had not bought in to the sink-or-swim bioethics. He performed the surgery immediately after my birth.

By the time I was 5, my surgeon, Dr. Lester Martin, had operated on me several dozen times. This is not unusual for children with my form of spina bifida (called myelomeningocele). It *was* unusual that I could walk, and did not have hydrocephalus (spinal fluid on the brain), which is standard for the condition. I did, however, have organ damage, an asymmetrical body, mobility problems and a limp. It was the beginning of a life among a chorus of strangers, all singing, *What's wrong with you? What's wrong with you?*

I coped by hiding myself inside a baggy wardrobe and a ferocious insistence that I was *normal.* I clung to the illusion that I was passing. I walked around without my glasses on (my myopia is impressive. So is the fact I was never run over) so that I'd never see my reflection in shop windows.

But nothing changes a disabled person's sense of self like another disabled person. I am a painter, and in 1995, I was invited to join a group of artists, writers and performers who were building disability culture. Their work was daring, edgy, funny and dark; it rejected old tropes that defined us as pathetic, frightening and worthless. They insisted that disability was an opportunity for creativity and resistance.

Growing up, I'd seen plenty of medical illustrations and freak show posters. The only images of the contemporary disabled body I'd ever seen were by photographers who used disabled subjects as avatars of psychological disturbance, such as found in the work of Joel-Peter Witkin. Creatures of suffering and sin. Monster imagery that taught me that I was a monster. I never saw work that depicted the beauty of disabled people, unless it was a trite and sappy form of beauty. (God preserve me from Inspiring Monuments to the Human Spirit.) With this new group, I was for the first time seeing disabled bodies as unexpected and charming and exciting. Each one stretched the boundaries of what it meant to be human. They made the world big enough to include me.

Today, as an adult, I am less than five feet tall. I have a curved spine. I wear huge, clunky orthopedic boots. I'm more visibly different than I've ever been—but I wear my glasses all the time now. My reflection doesn't cause me to flinch. I must say, it's nice not to collide with buildings, pedestrians, dogs and parked cars nearly as often.

The writer Elaine Scarry says in her book "On Beauty and Being Just" that beauty ignites in the viewer an urge to replicate. We wish to reproduce that which gives us aesthetic pleasure. The people I'd just met made me feel that impulse, as if I wanted to absorb who they were and recreate them as art. So, I swallowed and asked if I could do their portraits. They changed my life when they said yes.

I began by asking the collaborators about their careers and their personal lives. Portrait imagery was drawn from these conversations. I gave them a great deal of control over the images, because nearly all found it painful to be stared at, and I refused to replicate that pain. My collaborators claimed their own beauty in the process.

The deep aesthetic pleasure I feel can be explained through a single image. I first met poet, essayist and activist Eli Clare just before his gender transition. His portrait took two full years, during which I witnessed his metamorphosis. Eli's disability is cerebral palsy, which puts muscles under continuous isometric exercise. As a result, Eli's body is very defined, athletically "cut" in ways that are classically beautiful. In addition, Eli lives in Vermont, and is an avid hiker and cyclist. The way Eli uses his body, and the effect of his impairment gives him a grace woven of male and female ideals. Most people would never notice that a disability could be the direct cause of strength and health; yet this is the magical thing about bodies—they respond to the unexpected with their own forms of poetic genius.

I've been lucky to work with other prominent figures in disability culture, as well as members of the LGBTQ community, people who share histories of imposed stigma: the graphic novelist Alison Bechdel, author of "Fun Home" and "Are You My Mother?"; the British actor Mat Fraser, star of "American Horror Story: Freak Show;" Lynn Manning, a poet, playwright and founder of Watts Village Theater; Lennard Davis, a theorist of disability studies, whose memoirs recall his life as the hearing son of deaf parents; Nomy Lamm, a musician and activist around Fat and Queer identity; the psychologist, scholar and activist Rebecca Maskos, who is working to create a more vibrant disability culture in Germany; and the dancer Alice Sheppard, who helped redefine wheelchair-based choreography.

These portraits do not ask for sympathy, or empathy, or even that viewers agree that the subjects are beautiful. I simply want viewers to daydream the life of the person before them. To stretch ourselves toward a world where all bodies are exquisite, as they flow between all possible forms of what it is to be human.

I could easily have ended up as a teaching specimen in a jar. But luck gave me a surgeon. Fiery parents gave me a life outside of an institution. Today, I teach drawing in the Medical Humanities program at Northwestern University. My first- and second-year students draw the anomalous fetus collection in the cadaver lab. Each fetus has a different developmental impairment.

I teach my students to depict the specifics of every inch of the fetal bodies, until the drawings become profound examinations of bodies stopped in time. Their final assignment is to research a contemporary person with the same condition as their chosen fetus and do a presentation on his or her life. It helps these future doctors to stop seeing the specimens as historic artifacts or tragic medical problems. It's as if we're back at the Mutter, but this time those fetuses are given possible present lives, going forward in time.

I Lost My Voice, But Help Others Find Theirs

ALEX HUBBARD

I CAN TELL YOU THE EXACT MOMENT I REALIZED MY VOICE WAS BROKEN. I was sitting in a cubicle inside Pulitzer Hall, the home of the Columbia University Graduate School of Journalism. I was on the phone with a former top official at USA Hockey—a man whose name I knew well from having grown up a hockey fan. He was supposed to give me an interview for my master's project, a large journalism assignment that most other graduate students would compare to a thesis. I was excited for the help and also excited to speak to someone so well known to me. Then he said it.

"I'm sorry. I want to help you, but I can't understand you."

His words did not shock me; I had known for a long time that my voice was failing me. But what he said, with unintended cruel clarity, signaled to me that the moment had come. Later that day I—a 23-year-old Tennessee boy making good in New York City—called my mother and cried.

I was born in Nashville in the summer of 1990. A year later, it became clear to my parents that I could not see well, and by the time I was 2 years old, tests revealed that I was completely blind. As far as my family was concerned, this was of no matter. I was raised to think with no limits. For many years I attended public schools with sighted students, getting in trouble for the usual things like running in the halls. On my own decision, I began attending the state school for the blind when I was 11, where I played sports and graduated as the school's valedictorian.

When I was a senior in high school, a doctor noticed during a routine exam that my voice sounded abnormal to him. Further testing disclosed nine noncancerous tumors located on cranial nerves, which control almost everything about how the body's extremities work.

The diagnosis was neurofibromatosis Type 2, a disease caused by an inherited or spontaneous genetic mutation. About 100,000 Americans have one of the three forms of NF—NF Type 1, NF Type 2 or schwannomatosis, according to the National Institute of Neurological Disorders and Stroke. There is no cure, and extensive monitoring and treatment of individual symptoms is currently the recommended treatment.

The diagnosis was a shock, but it did not stop me from continuing my education. I went on to Middle Tennessee State University, where I served as both the sports and news editor of the school paper. I then became the first journalism student from my school to be admitted to the prestigious graduate program at Columbia and the first blind person to study in that program, according to institutional memories at both places. It was official: I was going to be a journalist.

My time at Columbia marked a great achievement for me, the first in my family to attend an Ivy League school, but it was also one of the darkest periods of my life. I had never considered merely being blind would prevent me from doing anything, but the tumors were slowly paralyzing my vocal cords and most of my tongue, sending my voice into a raspy spiral and making speech laborious. My college friends back in Tennessee had mostly met me when my throat was in much better shape, and as it worsened, they more or less grew accustomed to it as I did. But in New York I met people who clearly struggled to understand me and felt constricted by politeness and a well-meaning desire not to offend.

I avoided parties for fear they would be too loud. I stopped eating out because I couldn't eat much and was embarrassed that I might choke. I would sometimes sit for minutes at a time near someone I wanted to speak to, picking out the words I could best articulate, only to drop the whole plan and resign myself to silence.

I often overcame preconceptions about disability as a blind person with a sense of humor, but I soon discovered that when you are blind and then open your mouth to speak with a speech impediment, it is most likely that you are only confirming what they have already anticipated; you must have some deeper problem in the brain.

At Columbia, I began to experience a swift deterioration in my voice, or it seemed swift to me. During the school year, I had a minor surgery to try to increase my voice volume. In July 2014 after I graduated, I had a more involved surgery; that and a few other serious health complications knocked me flat for a while.

During this whole time I was searching for work. In October 2014 I began writing for The Contributor, Nashville's street paper, focusing on poverty, and then moved on to covering courts and legal affairs on a freelance basis for the Nashville Scene, an alt weekly. The entire time I just fought with my voice. I eventually gave up most phone use in favor of a relay-operator service, which allows me to type to an operator who speaks to the person on the line. It wasn't a perfect system, but it probably saved my career.

I had a great editor at the Scene, Jim Ridley, who was just an angel of a man. I was strongly considering hanging it up, applying for disability and hitting the couch. That's how discouraged I was when Jim came along. He didn't care anything about my health or any perceived limitations. He just wanted to see me write, and he trusted me without question.

Jim, who died in 2016, sustained my career long enough for the next opportunity to open up. A former professor let me know about a job at The Tennessean, a daily paper owned by Gannett. It was very simple, part-time work, mostly rewrite and handling letters to the editor. But they let me report some, and it grew into a full-time job.

Still, the deterioration of my voice was making reporting too difficult. So I asked to move behind the scenes. The request was one of the most painful things I have had to endure. Being a top-flight reporter was all I wanted to do.

I was given extra editing duties on the opinion page. Though it is not the same as chasing down breaking news, I have found that taking a piece of writing that may need a little guidance and seeing it shape up into a concise, informative column brings its own type of joy. I also occasionally get to write an opinion piece, which allows me to exercise my writing muscle and think critically.

I did make mistakes along the way. Concerned that my career would be affected if I revealed too much, and also not wanting to appear overly dramatic, I began withholding information about my health, even from people I loved and trusted. Doing this only created more questions in the minds of people who otherwise would have offered genuine support. Some of them fell away from me, and unable and unwilling to explain my plight, I let them go. I'm still recovering from this decision.

I am often told that I am an inspiration—usually because I hold down a job in a field not known for hosting very many disabled people. I appreciate what people mean by this, and honestly sometimes I'm surprised by it, too. But just as often I'm baffled by the complete separation between what I do for a living and the rest of my life.

I am not just a blind person who developed a severe speech impediment but didn't give up on his career dream. I am a young man with a quick wit, who is fluent in hockey, is widely read and can name every United States president in order, backward.

A doctor recently told me that my right vocal cord is out completely. This was not surprising. I suspect that it has probably been gone for as long as a year. Fortunately for me, and somewhat unusually, it hasn't collapsed, which is great news for my airway.

But it means that sometimes I'm not doing much more than whispering. There are good days and bad days for it; I have no insight into when they come and go.

But I have no plans to quit talking to you, so don't quit talking to me.

The "Madman" Is Back in the Building

ZACK McDERMOTT

WHAT DO YOU WEAR THE FIRST DAY BACK TO WORK AFTER A 90-day leave of absence because of a psychotic break? This is the question I found myself asking a little more than a year after I joined the Legal Aid Society of New York. The last time my colleagues had seen me, I'd been wearing a handlebar mustache better suited to a Hell's Angel than a 26-year-old public defender. I'd also taken to wearing a Mohawk—tried a case like that even. We won, thank God.

At the happy hour following that trial, I stripped down to my underwear and did a titillating strip tease for a bunch of law students who were there as a part of a recruiting event for a white shoe law firm. It didn't go over well but I didn't care. I thought I nailed it.

For my first day back to work I dressed in a sober navy sweater and a pair of dark slacks. Normal haircut, neatly trimmed beard. I got there early to avoid the morning rush and the inevitable stares and whispers. I had been "away with some issues"—that was the official company line, but offices are gossip hotbeds, and I wondered how much of the real story had filtered through. Did they know that I'd marched through the city for 12 hours—manic, psychotic and convinced I was being videotaped by secret TV producers, the star of my own reality show? That the police had found me later that evening shirtless, barefoot and crying on a subway platform? That I'd been involuntarily committed to Bellevue, the notorious psych ward to which we at Legal Aid routinely sent our most mentally ill clients?

For most, an involuntary stay in a locked psychiatric ward becomes a closely guarded secret. But part of me wanted everyone to know. I wanted them to know that I had received a Bipolar I diagnosis—that the "madman" they'd been covering for was actually a very sick young man who did things he feels guilty about, but who also knows that he had no more control over the doing of those things than a cancer patient has over the state of his lymph nodes.

Because that's the thing about mental illness—our brains betray us. Our symptoms are our behavior, and the disease makes us do humiliating and dangerous things.

In the weeks leading up to my break, I knew something was up with me. I couldn't sleep for more than a few hours each night, but seemed to have limitless reserves of energy. At times, I felt like electricity was shooting through my spine, that I was breathing in secrets of the universe.

I cried a lot, too. I'd listen to Bruce Springsteen sing "41 Shots" and weep in my room while I meditated on police brutality. These, I would learn, are all classic symptoms of bipolar disorder: the delusions of grandeur, the insomnia, the rapid cycling moods. And I was in my mid-20s—the textbook clinical age when bipolar disorder tends to present.

I wanted to tell my colleagues that the "madman"—the drunk, naked guy who ran through oncoming traffic and covered his wall in Sharpie—was gone. That he didn't go easy, that he had to be killed with a drug regimen that had left me drooling and impotent, with my hair falling out by the fistful, rapidly packing on weight.

Now I had to clean up the mess he'd made. The "madman" had raided my checking account, and there was no overdraft protection for "Sorry, I had a manic episode and rang up $800 worth of novelty T-shirts at Urban Outfitters." I'd lost friends, an apartment, maybe my job and reputation, too.

Mercifully, one person stuck by me through it all—my mom, nicknamed the Bird on account of the choppy, avian head movements she makes when her feathers are ruffled. She had been my tether in a hurricane.

During my leave of absence, I'd taken to calling the Bird in the middle of the night, every night, to hear her voice. I knew the toll it was taking on her. I could feel her heart breaking for me. She couldn't tell me that everything was going to be OK because the truth was, she wasn't sure. All she could do was make sure she kept answering the phone.

What I wanted to hear was, "This will never happen again." I wanted to hear that I'd never again be restrained and injected with antipsychotics. That I'd never have to smell that place again or eat that food. That I'd never again wonder if the orderlies would tackle the flailing patient before he *really* starts swinging. That I would never again fear the worst in a communal psych-ward shower. But no one, not even the Bird, could tell me that.

I buzzed my security card and entered the interior office. The halls of the Legal Aid Society felt nearly as claustrophobic as the psych ward. I wanted to believe that *these* people understood mental illness. They make their paltry living arguing on behalf of the poor and mentally ill, citing poverty and mental illness as an explanation for "bad" behavior every day in criminal court. But I was terrified of them.

I had to go talk to my supervisor. But just before I rounded the corner, my body made a U-turn back to the lobby and dove into the restroom. I fished my phone out of my pocket, scrolled to the Bs, and tapped Bird.

It was 8:30 a.m. in Kansas—she'd be busy setting up her students as they trickled into her class. She answered on the first ring; her phone had become an appendage since I moved back to New York.

"Gorilla report?" (The Bird nicknamed me Gorilla, because of my barrel chest and hirsute body.)

"Gorilla is at Legal Aid."

"First day of school? Not good?"

"Not good." I spilled it—sobbed, breathed, sobbed. "I shouldn't be here. This is so ridiculous. I feel like such an idiot. Idiot! I can't see these people again yet."

"Steppers keep on stepping. You're a . . ."

"Not a stepper! Not a stepper. No steps."

"Three months ago you were in a locked psych ward. You're at work now. You're still an attorney. It's not easy, what you're doing."

"I'm scared. Of everyone. And everything—all the time," I told her. "The subway. Confined spaces. Walking through the halls, waiting for everyone to stare at me, and think, The Madman is back in the building."

"You need Mama Gorilla to open up five cans of whoop ass on somebody?"

I laughed. I knew she'd love to.

"Boy, we been through the fire with gasoline soaked drawers on. You got this. Puff out that big gorilla chest and go rip it off like a Band-Aid. Call me if you need me."

I wiped my eyes, left the stall, and splashed some cold water on my face. Game time. *Don't let them see you sweat. Steppers keep on stepping.* I looked in the mirror—*You look good, you look normal. You're a normal guy.* Then I slapped myself in the face as hard as I could.

I knew I had a lifelong disease and that bipolar disorder is something to be managed, not cured. I knew I'd need to take medication for the rest of my life and that I'd humiliated myself in front of countless friends and strangers alike. I knew that I had more in common than I'd have liked with my schizophrenic uncle Eddie who lived the last 15 years of his life in a state mental institution. That no matter how early I got to work, no matter how useful I made myself, no matter how reasonable and modest my khakis and my sweater were, I was and would always be the "crazy" dude.

I finally bucked up and made it to my supervisor's office. I knew we'd have a come-to-Jesus talk soon enough—my practice was in disarray when I left—but he seemed genuinely glad to see me. "You look great," he told me. "Got some meat back on your bones. We're thrilled to have you back."

Twenty minutes later, he was forced to dismiss me. I needed a note from my psychiatrist declaring me fit to return to duty. "Sorry," he said, "it's just policy. You can't be in the building without a note."

"Them's the rules," I said.

I was relieved to have an out but I was humiliated all the same. The note requirement didn't feel like the fulfillment of a bureaucratic requirement; it felt like a request for proof of sanity. *We're thrilled to have you. Now we'll be needing certification that you're no longer certifiable.*

I got the note the next day and returned. I knew I had no choice but to keep showing up every day, take my meds, keep my pants on and channel my trauma as best I could to find a way to be someone else's Bird.

It did not work.

What I'd once viewed as my dream job became a pressure cooker I couldn't withstand. The cramped jail cells where we public defenders spend so much of our working day frequently triggered PTSD symptoms, bringing me right back to the claustrophobia of forced confinement. But it was the anxiety attacks *after* work that eventually did me in. My philosophy as a public defender was that no one should spend an extra hour in jail because of a mistake I made. It's probably an impossible standard to meet, but I couldn't shake the fear that I wasn't cutting it. After two more psychotic breaks and hospitalizations, I left the Legal Aid Society.

It's been two years now, and thanks to the love and support of the Bird and modern pharmacology, I no longer live in constant fear that my mind will abandon me at any time. I also live with the knowledge that millions of others with mental illness live with that fear, and suffer through it alone, and far too many are sucked into our hyperactive justice system and treated as criminals for an illness they are powerless to fight. A 2015 investigation by The Times found that nearly 40 percent of the population at Rikers Island, a total of 4,000 men and women at any given time, suffer from mental illness. In other words, our jails have become our de facto mental health facilities.

Ultimately, I couldn't take the pressure of having lives hanging in the balance when I went off to work in the morning, while also keeping my bipolar in check.

What I could do, though, was speak and write honestly about being utterly at the mercy of my illness, and being pulled from the brink by the care of one person's love. And that's what I am doing now.

Hildegard's Visions, and Mine

JENNY GIERING

I DON'T KNOW WHY I DIDN'T JUST TURN THE CAR AROUND AND GO HOME. Perhaps I didn't want to face failure again, unable to complete even the simplest of mom tasks—driving my son to his hockey game.

The morning had already been harder than it should have been: my joints achier, the car door heavier, the mid-December chill sharper in my lungs. I blasted the heater as we pulled out of the driveway and headed down the hill toward town. I swerved, barely missing a mailbox, trying to navigate through a six-inch square of frost-free glass. I pushed buttons, changed settings, convinced the heater wasn't working properly. *Why was it taking so long to clear the ice?* I hurled a stream of invective so furious it was met with silence from my son in the back seat—until he replied in a tiny, quiet voice, "Mommy, you only turned on the heater, like, two seconds ago."

That was my first clue that something strange was happening in my brain. Those seconds had stretched into vast, immeasurable time. Now, my chest burned. I rounded a corner, shifted my gaze from the dashboard to the road, and my peripheral vision danced with neon snowflakes. The familiar, rural landscape suddenly appeared in hyper 3-D, as if I were looking through a child's View-Master. I wondered if I'd taken my morning meds twice.

Whatever was happening, this high-gloss, Technicolor world was not something of my own design. I couldn't focus on the road or my son's voice chiming in from the back seat. My mind bucked every effort to corral it by backing itself into rooms deep in my consciousness. I had no idea what was happening, but I kept driving.

Through a precarious combination of luck and foolishness, we made it to the rink safely, but as I sat in the lobby, heart racing, intensely dizzy and disoriented, I handed my phone to a stranger and asked him to call 911.

That first spell lasted seven hours. The hospital treated me for a migraine and sent me home with a diagnosis of fatigue. After that, the spells came every day, sometimes more than once. If they happened while I was sleeping, I would wake up, chest burning, hearing dogs walking around the bed or a chorus of tropical birds. I watched the ceiling liquefy. Purple henna designs scrolled across my vision like a news crawl on TV. I stopped driving. I stopped leaving the house. We tried to identify the cause, but the spells refused to conform to a pattern. And nothing helped.

For weeks, I toggled between these dissociative hallucinatory states and blinding, raging head pain. I spent three days in a neurological unit in Boston, hoping for answers. But the test results followed a familiar pattern: My brain was fine, but clearly I was not.

In the end, my doctors gave me an enormous stress dose of steroids to break the migraine cycle. But the night the headache broke, I had the strongest spell of all.

My mind cleaved. I saw my thoughts pour out in a scrambled, encrypted wave that crested just beyond the back of my head. I was convinced that if I could decipher their code, I would unlock an artistic secret, a creative message.

I've been thinking a lot lately about Hildegard von Bingen, the 12th-century composer, abbess, inventor and saint. Like me, she suffered from chronically poor health. The neurologist Oliver Sacks retroactively diagnosed her condition as intractable migraines. Hildegard also had elaborate visions; this would make sense if Dr. Sacks's diagnosis was correct. Some migraines are accompanied by elaborate and detailed hallucinations. In a theological work, "Scivias," she described an experience strikingly similar to my own:

"When I was 42 years and 7 months old, Heaven was opened and a fiery light of exceeding brilliance came and permeated my whole brain, and inflamed my whole heart and my whole breast."

Hildegard is best known, though, for her music—a powerful body of mystical religious chants that are listened to more widely today than the music of any other single composer of her time.

I want to talk to her.

Before I got sick, I was a productive theater composer. I was a mom and a wife, a multitasker and an overachiever. I wrung every bit of usable time from my days. Anything I accomplish now gets done through a haze of illness. There are fleeting moments when inspiration converges with a stretch of good days or when, through sheer force of will, I can make myself focus long enough to bring a song into the world. Those are rare days.

I wonder what Hildegard would tell me. Somehow, she turned her mystical visions into transcendent madrigals. What alchemy did she use to marry her debility to inspiration?

A couple of months before the incident with my son in the car, Social Security had declared me disabled, after a three-year battle with an autoimmune syndrome born from a toxic reaction to the silicone implant I had received during a mastectomy. Sometimes my symptoms are tolerable. Other times, I careen into crisis, the consequence of a hair-trigger immune system: the loss of more than a third of my body weight; the persistent infection that took seven rounds of antibiotics to clear; the bout of norovirus so severe my husband had to carry me into the emergency room. Every cough, every twinge of nausea can tip over into bad health from which I take months to recover. Like a masked marauder, my illness creeps into different bodily systems, wreaking havoc. I never know what's next.

I don't have Hildegard's faith, nor do I believe things happen for a reason. I certainly don't attach any higher meaning to my illness. I know in my heart only that a confluence of then-unknown factors and bad luck has brought me to the barracks of ill health. But

I can't stop thinking about these strange spells. What mark will they have on my music? And do I have a responsibility to decipher them as a road map? Or a warning?

I asked my husband this as I lay hallucinating in bed next to him. Gently, he demurred, saying he didn't know.

A year into my illness, I started writing songs about my experience. Like live tweets of a tragedy, they are real-time snapshots of a life gone off the rails—a woman constantly redefined into smaller and smaller boxes. What I want this piece of theater to communicate has morphed radically since I lived through these months of altered consciousness. I just don't know what it is yet.

These days, the spells are less dramatic, but ever-present, like my own personal background radiation, punctuated by deafening tinnitus, pressure, pain and heat, like a fire behind the door of my eyes. My six doctors are uncertain of the cause, leaving me wondering if this is forever.

Disability has forced me to master the art of changing expectations. I have to live in the constantly shifting landscape of my illness. Every plan, every dinner date, every trip comes with the proviso that I may not be up to the task. Sometimes all I can do is let go.

One thing, however, is definite: These spells have given me a renewed sense of purpose. I am acutely aware that I need to get as much music out of my pen while I am able. I know that the next medical crisis will come. When it does, I know it will set me back weeks, if not months. Illness is baked into me now. Perhaps this is what Hildegard knew: Say what you can, as well as you can, for as long as you can.

Finding Myself on the Page

ONA GRITZ

ONE MORNING IN MY 18TH SUMMER, THE GUY I THOUGHT I LOVED stopped by to invite my roommates and me to pick apricots from the tree he'd discovered behind the Boulder Public Library. Five of us gathered paper grocery sacks and trooped over, marveling that in the several weeks we'd all been in town, studying poetry at Naropa Institute, none of us had noticed the fruit tree. Actually, the others marveled and I pretended to. Growing up in Queens, N.Y., the only apricots I'd seen came dried and flattened into sticky sheets on paper backing my mother bought in rolls.

My friends that summer were all older, worldlier and better read than I. Happily, I slipped into the role they offered—protégé and favored little sister. They critiqued my poems and presented me with reading lists. The women among them gave me relationship advice, but we hadn't discussed what had happened the night before at a classmate's backyard party: Rich had finally kissed me.

"Catch," he called now from atop the tree and tossed down what looked like miniature peaches. I lifted my Indian print skirt to form a net as two thoughts vied for my attention. *Maybe he could love me. I need to write about this.*

Nothing ever came of my infatuation with Rich. Nor did anything come of my attempts to capture that perfect summer morning in a poem, despite that, to my teenage sensibilities, it had all the right ingredients. Longing, hope, a cute guy with a twisted front tooth, those apricots dropping softly.

The problem was that I didn't have much to say about the experience other than that it felt important to me. Then one day, more than 20 years later, an image came to me of my younger self poised beneath that tree and I realized what was missing from those early drafts. My cerebral palsy.

Back on that July morning in 1981, the moment my crush told my new friends and me of his finding, my mind raced. I'd stay in my impractical, wraparound skirt. This would give me an excuse to wait below while the others, dressed in shorts and sneakers, performed the impossible feat of climbing the tree. Once there, I made another split-second decision to lift my skirt and expose my mismatched calves. It was either that or admit that I couldn't catch anything more challenging than a balloon in my clumsy hands.

Calculations of this kind were second nature to me. By the time I had language, I'd made an unspoken pact with nearly everyone I encountered. *I won't talk about my body's awkwardness and limitations and neither will you.*

"What happened to your leg?"

I hated when the pact was broken with questions like that. In grade school, I usually went with the clipped but accurate "Nothing." After all, whatever caused my cerebral palsy occurred long before, during my birth. Also, it didn't happen to my leg, but to the part of my brain that tells that leg to move.

Once, in sixth grade, a friend whispered that another classmate posed the question to her. "I said you fell off the Empire State Building." "And she believed you?" "I don't know, but she changed the subject."

After that, I told that 1,250-foot tall tale a few times myself. Though I'd stolen it, it seemed like a more original and interesting version of my other standby, "None of your beeswax."

My form of cerebral palsy, right hemiplegia, includes among its symptoms numbness along one side of my body. When, at 5 years old, I asked my own first question about it, "Why do I feel more on the left?" my mother had an answer ready. Only it wasn't an answer at all.

"Because your heart is on the left," she said. "Like everyone's."

This memory is clear to me, but there must have been times before that when my parents talked to me about my disability. After all, I knew what I had and what it was called. Cerebral, a long C word like "carnival." Palsy, which sounded a little like "pansy." My disability had a nickname, C.P., and it was why I had to wear a leg brace to bed and visit a physical therapist once a month at a place my parents referred to as the Center.

"It's nothing, barely noticeable," my mother assured me as she helped me with my leg brace at night. I knew she was right, at least compared with some of the kids I saw at the Center whose C.P. was so bad they made strange grunts when they tried to talk and couldn't walk at all. At the same time, I knew we were alike, those kids and I, in some deep, undeniable way. The only thing that separated us was luck, a tiny L word that, like "life" and "love," was somehow big enough to make all the difference in the world.

As a child trying to understand something about living in my body and in our community, neither of my mother's explanations was of much use. I don't say this to fault my mother. She grew up, as most of us did, being told not to point or to stare or to ask questions when it came to ways that people differ. This is where that pact of silence originates, from our attempt to be thoughtful and careful with one another. Now more than ever, while the emotionally delayed bully who inhabits our highest office models baiting, cruelty and mockery instead, every attempt at kindness is essential.

But where does that leave me, and others like me, as we tiptoe around the sensitive subject of our otherness? For a long time, I felt unsure not only of how to talk about my disability but even how to think about it. Its meaning was slippery and ever-changing. When I was little it meant I couldn't roller skate or run like the other kids. In my teens and early 20s, it was the flaw that made me less attractive than my friends. When, at 25, I became involved with a handsome, able, but very difficult man, disability was the scrim through which he looked like my one chance at love.

We married and had a child, and as I struggled with the physically demanding tasks involved in caring for a newborn, my disability revealed itself for what it was all along—a set of specific limitations that required modifications, creativity and, more often than I was comfortable with, that I ask for help. That first year of parenting was among the hardest I've lived through, and the most humbling. At the same time, it was what finally led me into an authentic relationship with my body, one based on what I needed to accomplish rather than how I was perceived.

Through it all, I was writing. But it would be several more years before I began to explore disability in my work.

What am I trying to say? What is this poem, essay, chapter about? What details belong in the piece and what's extraneous? These are among the questions all writers ask ourselves as we stare at the blinking cursors on our computer screens. When it comes to how relevant my cerebral palsy is to a given piece, the question can seem even more complex.

"Would I have to be disabled on every page?" I asked a friend who is also a literary agent when she suggested I write a memoir on mothering with a disability. The question, in its muddled state, made us laugh. But what I was trying to ascertain was whether the narrator—the "me" on the page—had to be thinking about cerebral palsy in every scene of her story when, in life, this was far from true.

Over time I discovered a more useful line of inquiry as I wrote. *Would details about my disability not only expand this passage but also deepen it? Would they bring forth something I'd yet to articulate, perhaps didn't even know I knew?*

The page is where I finally came to understand my own body and its evolving narrative, where I continue to learn when my disability informs a particular dynamic and when it's beside the point. Eventually, I rewrote the poem about the morning of the apricots, and it was only then that I realized how lonely I'd been, even among friends I nearly worshiped. After all, there was this important aspect not just of my experience, but of my very being, that I didn't think I could share with anyone.

"Do something with your brokenness," David Hernandez urges in his poem "Sincerely, the Sky."

It's a call to all of us, since everyone is broken in places if we're to tell the whole story. And especially in these factious times, telling the whole of our stories, whether on the page or in the flesh, gives us the best chance we have to truly connect.

Should I Tell My Students I Have Depression?

ABBY L. WILKERSON

THE NEW CLASS I WAS TEACHING—"COMPOSING DISABILITY: CRIP Ecologies"—was one of several first-year writing seminars offered at George Washington University. Given the focus, it was likely to be a challenge for at least some of the students. And it was presenting a particular challenge to me.

Even before the class began, I was anxious. I have depression, and I wondered: Should I acknowledge it in the class? Would the students benefit if I did? I wanted to be sure I knew what I was doing, for everyone's sake, before taking the leap. But I was not at all certain. The idea of disclosing in the classroom made me feel conflicted and vulnerable.

Though the World Health Organization identifies depression as "the leading cause of disability," not everyone with depression identifies herself as disabled. One of the central meanings of disability for me is "crip" pride—resistance to medical notions of disability as a defect and related social stigmas. My depression has given me unasked-for gifts, including a sensitivity to others' suffering.

But let's face it—on some level, depression *is* suffering. How could I reconcile this with the fierce crip attitude in others that I've so admired? In class, how would the dull weight of depression sit with the "crip" in the course title? If I were going to do this, I needed to get it right. And I wasn't sure how.

Though I have suffered severe depression in the past, these days, my episodes tend to be milder and less frequent. Some days, I feel fine. But I might soon begin feeling melancholy—yet still able to laugh, think clearly, sleep at night and enjoy my life. Then one morning, for no discernible reason, I wake up mired in mud, my body now freight to be pushed through daily routines. The rhythm of life is suddenly ground down almost to nothing. I feel somehow both numb and raw, skin thin, laid open. Everything that matters is now far-off in the distance. Other people seem remote, existing in some parallel universe.

I always have to be learning how to take better care of myself, noticing signs of a depression emerging, yet I also have to accept depression as part of me. I'd need to continue these efforts while teaching a new course posing heightened emotional demands for students, on a campus where several of their peers had committed suicide over the previous year or so.

At the first class I asked the students to write about a time when they or someone close to them had become vulnerable. I did not mention my depression. When they returned for the next class I asked how the writing had gone. A few students exchanged glances. Then one, a young man, said, a bit eagerly, a bit nervously: "It was hard to know what to write about! We had to decide how vulnerable to make ourselves to a roomful of people we don't even know." His classmates laughed in recognition, and soon several people were speaking at once.

The feminist philosopher Marilyn Frye contends that double-bind situations are routine for members of oppressed groups. Though she didn't apply this claim to disability, it certainly fits. Whether or not to disclose depression is a classic double bind. Disclose, and face stigma, and perhaps material repercussions. Don't disclose, and your suffering may remain invisible, you may face judgments about your character when depression alters your affect and behavior, and you remain isolated. (As I once heard a cashier intone sadly to another customer in what instantly became known to me as The Drugstore of Existential Despair, "No one can help you.") In silence, you are unable to explicitly draw on your own experience of depression to help or connect with others in the same situation.

At times when one's depression is not acute, it's easy to feel there's no need to disclose; and when it is, it can seem unthinkable. My past disclosures have been fairly limited. In an academic context, disclosing has particular nuances, for students and faculty members alike. Rationality is the key to functioning in an academic setting; being smooth and continually productive is the basic requirement for survival. Mental illness doesn't fit into that picture.

Part way into the semester, we were discussing Allie Brosh's depression narrative in "Hyperbole and a Half." She describes people trying to help her with "hope-centric" talk, and her inability to convey to them that this approach simply doesn't compute when one is severely depressed. One of my students spoke up with more than a little anger: "If one of my friends acts depressed, how can I not try to cheer them up?" he asked. "The author talks like it's wrong to want to help somebody I care about. It's like there's no right thing to do."

An uncharacteristic silence fell.

He added, more softly: "But I'm not the kind of guy to get depressed. Maybe I just don't understand these things."

Then another student began to speak; she matter-of-factly told us about her chronic anxiety and fears of telling others about it, something we'd never heard from her. Yet another spoke up for the first time about his depression: "Just let the person talk," he said. "That's big. Most people don't want to hear about it. That's what she's saying. They just want you to cheer up when that's the one thing you can't do."

Suddenly the work of the class took on new energy. Part of their coursework involved conducting interviews with other students on campus—about depression and anxiety in LGBTQ students, about learning disabilities, about sports injuries in athletes, and more. A group of students presented their results at the George Washington University conference, Composing Disability: Crip Ecologies.

(This conference had been one of my inspirations for creating the new course.) All of them had begun to discover for themselves what we'd been reading about—how social environments structure our experiences of disability. The following weeks amounted to a sustained response to the conversation cracked open by that small but honest expression of frustration.

Meanwhile, the unsettled feeling lingered in the pit of my stomach. I never disclosed my depression in class. And I am still not sure why.

Professors are beginning to tell their stories, and to acknowledge what's at stake for us in disclosing mental disability. Those in contingent positions (nontenured, nontenure track—now the majority of all faculty appointments in the United States) particularly fear the consequences of disclosure. They could be perceived differently, affecting student course evaluations or peer and administrator assessments, effects that are likely to be compounded for women, people of color, LGBTQ, or older people. Fears of problems with health insurance are not unreasonable.

I'm relatively lucky in my own contingent appointment. The position is "indefinitely renewable" with a livable salary and full benefits, and I was able to apply for promotion to associate professor (and succeed). These conditions are vastly better than those faced by most contingent faculty members. Renewable is good. But indefinite is, well, definitely not definite.

Perhaps the professor's job isn't always to profess. Sometimes it's making way for the not-so-small miracle of thinking together to burst open—and be taken up again and again.

Sandie Friedman, a friend I teach with who also has depression, once wrote, "I remind myself every morning that it is enough to swim through the day, even in the slow lane—doing the things you don't want to do, being visible when you would prefer not to be. That already is a lot."

When my students made their own vulnerabilities apparent, they were doing a lot, like Sandie swimming every day. Their example has encouraged me to engage in these reflections here and now, and to determine appropriate ways to acknowledge my depression in future courses. At my students' age, knowing a professor with the same struggle might have made my depression a little more . . . thinkable, compatible with a rich and meaningful life, less my personal failing. How do we loosen the double bind and remove the fear of risking careers and relationships? Sometimes vulnerability loves—and needs—company.

We Are the Original
Lifehackers

LIZ JACKSON

IT WAS 1988 WHEN BETSEY FARBER FOUND HERSELF HACKING THROUGH A dried-up nest of wild thyme in the backyard of a rental home in Provence. The scene was aromatic and picturesque, except for the pair of children's scissors she'd stuffed her grown-up knuckles through. She couldn't find anything better for the job. *Who is going to leave their good kitchen tools in a rental?* She had just finished disassembling an unbudging pepper grinder, soaking the rusted metal parts in a glass of Coca-Cola so she could season dinner.

Betsey and her husband, Sam, began to scour local hardware stores and weekend markets for better kitchen tools. But kitchen supply offerings were limited to slender, pointed, gripless products. What Betsey was hoping to find were more like the hand tools that New England Shakers had crafted a century before, with their beautifully and purposeful tactile handles. Sam, who had started a successful housewares business in 1960, began to plan a new line of kitchen tools with Betsey that would feel good, not just in her hand but in anyone's hand. That was the genesis of the cooking tools and housewares company OXO, established in 1990.

Since then OXO has become a nearly universal example of universal design, a concept that strives to produce products and spaces accessible to everyone, disabled or not. It produces more than 1,000 products sold globally.

But in learning about Betsey and OXO, something caught my eye. This is from the OXO Blog: "Sam Farber founded OXO when he saw his wife, Betsey, having trouble holding her peeler due to arthritis. This got Sam thinking: Why do ordinary kitchen tools hurt your hands? Sam saw an opportunity to create more thoughtful cooking tools that would benefit all people (with or without arthritis) and promised Betsey he would make a better peeler."

As a disabled designer, I have come to believe that products are a manifestation of relationships. Disabled people have long been integral to design processes, though we're frequently viewed as "inspiration" rather than active participants. When I discovered Betsey was a talented architect in her own right, I began to wonder about her relationship to OXO. And so I reached out to ask.

When Betsey and I finally met, we quickly began doing exactly what my disabled friends and I do—we shared our life hacks, the creative ways we alter things to make them more accessible. I told her about the dancer and writer Jerron Herman who orders a pizza cutter with his waffle at the local diner, which works much better for him than a knife and fork, and Emily Ladau who uses kitchen tongs to extend her reach. Betsey told me about the time she wired the jar opener that was affixed to the bottom of her cabinet to a cheese grater so she could hold it in her hand. When Betsey and Sam sold OXO in 1996, the OXO Good Grips Jar Opener was their No. 2 product, second only to their peeler.

Our conversation left me wondering when a hack becomes more than a hack and turns into something of commercial value. And moreover, I wanted to know why these inventions aren't routinely written into disability history.

Such stories reach back centuries and continue on to the present day, but they often go untold. For instance, you probably have not heard of Stephan Farffler, the Nuremberg-based watchmaker and paraplegic who in 1655 created what he called the manumotive carriage. Farffler accomplished two things with his invention; he created the first self-propelled wheelchair, and unbeknown to him, it became the precursor for the modern-day bicycle.

Today, the technologies we use often come from people like

Wayne Westerman, who as an electrical engineering doctoral student at the University of Delaware in the late 1990s was experiencing symptoms of repetitive stress syndrome that interfered with his ability to study and work. With his adviser John Elias, he went on to help develop touch-screen technologies and establish a company called FingerWorks, which would pave the way for the tablet and cellphone revolution that shapes most of our lives today. If you are reading this piece on your phone right now, you may want to thank Westerman. Steve Jobs bought FingerWorks in 2005, and it led to the iPhone touch screen.

These stories exemplify what it means to be an original life-hacker; our unique experiences and insights enable us to use what's available to make things accessible. Yet, despite this history of creating elegant solutions for ourselves, our contributions are often overshadowed or misrepresented, favoring instead a story with a savior as its protagonist.

This was the case with OXO. "The general understanding," Betsey told me, "was of the brilliance and kindness of Sam who made these tools for his poor crippled wife so she could function in the kitchen. I will probably go down in history as having arthritis rather than having the conceptual idea of making these comfortable for your hand."

This predominant narrative that disabled people are only recipients of design has managed to embed itself into our language. The phrase "design *for* disability" yields many more Google search results than "disability design." OXO may think its handle fixes us, but I see the lack of attribution as the disabling issue.

When people like Betsey take credit for their contributions, it allows someone like me to take ownership of mine. This is how we attract disabled people to design.

Betsey now lives in what she calls an elder community. A group of designers recently asked her and a few of her neighbors to test a gripping tool prototype. As Betsey was trying it out, she thought of her OXO Jar Opener and told the designers, "You know, if you put the grip on one side instead of both, it will be lighter and more efficient." They took her advice. I asked Betsey if they had any idea who she was. Laughing, she said no.

It is my hope that they know now, and that one day everyone will know what we do.

IV

NAVIGATING

My Supercharged, Tricked Out, Bluetooth Wheelchair Life Force

KATIE SAVIN

My BEST ROUTE 88 AC TRANSIT FRIEND HAS CANCER. HE'S WAITING until the end of the holidays to "turn himself in" to the hospital, where they'll "poke him all over," but he knows in any case he has to do this soon because there's a big lump on his stomach. I didn't know how much I'd begun to care for him, my fellow in-a-wheelchair bus rider, until I felt my sadness become a different kind of lump in my throat.

My friend Olantis and his chair, Roscoe, emit more life than I've seen from any walkie. He tricked out Roscoe with some seriously powerful Bluetooth speakers through which he blasts the music that matches his mood—sometimes gospel, sometimes house, usually something with a good beat and lyrics that make you think. Olantis is big. He's tall and fat. He's black. His voice booms and his laugh ricochets. He goes so fast in Roscoe! The first time I saw him, before we'd officially met, he was zooming down Shattuck Avenue weaving in and out of groups of students walking in clusters with their oversized backpacks. His music was blasting. This man was up in every available sensory input of every single passer-by.

I wasn't envious just that Roscoe had the horsepower to go so much faster than Anita (my own motorized wheelchair). I was also envious of Olantis's flagrant disregard of social norms. I spend my days at Cal trying to balance my need to advocate my right to physically enter spaces with my perceived need to not offend anyone in the process—by dressing modestly, not too dykey, careful not to break any obvious gender or fashion rules; by keeping my mouth shut in the face of minor issues if I can deal with them on my own; by projecting a friendly and helpful attitude as much as I can. It doesn't always work, though, so seeing and being with Olantis is sometimes liberating.

I make the two-mile commute most weekdays to fulfill my duties as a doctoral student at the University of California, Berkeley—to attend class, work as a teaching assistant, research or go to meetings. Anita helps me from home to school and in and out of the buildings on campus as I deal with my collection of conditions—asthma, Type 1 diabetes, Ehlers-Danlos syndrome and dysautonomia among them. Anita allows me to stay in the game and remain competitive as a student and teacher, despite the daily exclusions and presumptions of incompetence I face. I've learned to thicken my skin and employ my stubborn nature. But the connections I make with other disabled people like Olantis along the way help keep me going in ways Anita can't.

Olantis sells papers, the kind that homeless people sell for a dollar each. He has to collect them between 5 and 7 a.m. at the pickup point, and his pain has been worse recently, so he hasn't been able to go to sleep until 2 or 3 a.m. and he simply can't get up in time. "I sell papers," he said. "That's who I am. I'm nothing without my hustle." He continued on about feeling depressed and concerned about finances. This was our somber discussion that day on the 88 bus, which, like all the others, started at the beginning of the line. The conversation in which he told me he had cancer.

The first time we talked, we were in the long line of people waiting for the bus. There was hip-hop booming out of the back of Roscoe. I was absent-mindedly bopping along to it while I exhaled my long day and relaxed into the beat, enjoying the pieces of my old life filled with dancing that I could still hold onto. He asked me if I liked it. I said yes, I love your music, and asked him how he had affixed the speakers to his chair. I showed off my cellphone and USB chargers that I had affixed to my chair, purely for bragging rights (Olantis was impressed). Then, eternally endearing himself to my inner 10-year-old boy, he asked if I wanted to race.

"I've seen you zoom down Shattuck!" I yelped. "I know you're gonna win!" I don't like to lose. He laughed and relished in the moment of my admitting defeat pre-race and asked to see me and Anita go at top speed. This is my kind of waiting-for-the-bus activity. So Anita and I went at it with all our might as he looked on laughing, saying, "Come on, that's it?"

I enter another space in a wheelchair, one in which the homeless and disabled people like Olantis are quick to greet me and talk to me while the able-bodied world averts its gaze. Even with my disability, I realize I am in a place of privilege—a white, middle-class woman pursuing a doctorate, with access to medical insurance. I know that Olantis does not share this privilege. I know that I am lucky to be in the space I am at Berkeley, but the challenges it brings can be emotionally draining and painful. My time with Olantis is anything but. The crip-bus-bond isn't just tolerant; it's fully embracing of me, *because* of my cripness, not in spite of it.

I love the world Olantis and Roscoe and Anita and I have created in our exile, where we are free to call our wheelchairs by name and bop to the music. Where we giggle too easily at the slightest perception of innuendo. Where we drag race and brag about getting first-class seats since the bus driver loads the wheelchairs first.

I hope Olantis survives his stomach cancer. I would really, really miss our fun evening commutes. I want to offer to get his papers at 5 a.m. so that he can keep selling them, but I know I'm too crip to do that, so I'll have to just listen and empathize, sit face to face with the truth that disability and poverty are intertwined, and understand how painful it is when we feel our bodies no longer able to carry out the activities that sustain us.

Olantis, if I make it longer than you do in this world that was never designed for us, if I'm still ignoring the haters who tell us we slow down their commute and you're not beside me, I hereby promise, I'll hook up Anita with Bluetooth speakers. We won't be invisible, or silent, with you and Roscoe as our supercharged, tricked out sensory-power life force.

New York Has a Great Subway, If You're Not in a Wheelchair

SASHA BLAIR-GOLDENSOHN

O N A BRIGHT SUMMER MORNING IN MANHATTAN IN 2009, I WAS WALK-ing through Central Park when an enormous rotted tree branch snapped and fell on my head.

What came next was a remarkable turn of events that saved my life. First, a doctor out for a morning jog saw me lying unconscious, and used a pair of jeans he dug out of my backpack to slow the bleeding until an ambulance came. I was treated at the intensive care unit at NewYork-Presbyterian Hospital and underwent rehabilitation at Helen Hayes Hospital in Rockland County, where a skilled medical team worked tirelessly for more than a month treating injuries to my head, lungs and spine. And over the next six months, nonstop support from loved ones and expert rehabilitative care helped me recover much of what I had lost.

But there was one feat they could not accomplish. The accident had caused spinal cord damage, which partly paralyzed my lower body. It was clear I was going to have to use a wheelchair to get around.

Among the first challenges I faced was navigating my neighborhood in New York on wheels. With practice, I slowly increased my range, and began getting around the city independently. I took buses, taxis and eventually the subway. I returned to work as a software engineer at Google 18 months after my accident.

I felt grateful to have come back so far, but each time a broken curb tipped over my wheelchair, a taxi refused to stop for me or a stalled subway elevator left me stranded, my frustration mounted. I became increasingly aware of how large, inflexible bureaucracies with a "good enough" approach to infrastructure and services can disenfranchise citizens with disabilities, many of whom cannot bridge these gaps on their own.

Before my injury, I had felt that dealing with grittiness and unreliability were the price of entry for living in New York, and even took a smug pride in dealing with obstacles. Since my accident, I have been humbled to realize the often dire effect of civic dysfunction on the vulnerable, and have had to recognize that some of what I once took for resourcefulness was in truth enabled by privilege.

I was once like many other able-bodied New Yorkers, only vaguely aware of subway elevators, merely noting that they seemed dingy and often out of service. But now that I needed them, the reality was more stark. New York's subway is by far the least wheelchair-friendly public transit system of any major American city, with fewer than 100 of the system's 425 stations accessible. That means fewer than one in four stations can be used by people in wheelchairs when elevators are working—and they frequently are not.

On average, 25 elevators a day stop working, and these breakdowns are not quickly resolved; their median duration is nearly four hours. Moreover, with a single elevator serving both directions at most stops, a breakdown means that a disabled rider exiting the train will be trapped on the platform, and one hoping to board will have to find some other way to travel to where they need to go.

Other problems make this bad situation worse: There is no sure way for riders to know when a breakdown has occurred: There are no intercom announcements, and the listings on the Metropolitan Transportation Authority's website are unreliable. In the past month only two of the eight elevator failures I encountered were listed, making it likely that official statistics are an undercount.

I often wheel off a train only to discover that the sole elevator to ground level is out of service. No information on alternate routes is posted as it is for other service changes and delays—indeed, subway personnel are often unaware of the situation. So the options are to wait for the next train and continue to an accessible stop— possibly many stations away—or call the fire department to be carried up the stairs.

I've done both, although on occasion fellow passengers have agreed to carry me—a 170-pound stranger in a wheelchair—up to the street. And it has been heartening to find that in moments of need, people step forward to help.

But these acts by individuals cannot be accepted as a substitute for a functional system. Rather, a system that routinely leaves vulnerable riders stranded has abdicated its responsibility. The need for extraordinary goodness, like that shown by the doctor in Central Park, should be the exception, not the rule.

All of this can make an accessible subway seem impossible. But it isn't.

When I traveled to Boston several years ago, I was amazed to discover that its subway system—as old as New York's, though far smaller, with only 53 stations—is more than 90 percent wheelchair accessible.

Was Boston just a nicer town? Not necessarily. The admirable accessibility was legally mandated. In 2002, wheelchair users sued Boston's transit authority and the eventual settlement included guarantees for elevator construction, maintenance and monitoring.

So are legal challenges the only way to get equal access for the disabled? They are undoubtedly a useful tool, and sometimes a necessary one. But however change comes, accessibility advocates will have to counter the belief that devoting resources to help one group necessarily shortchanges others.

The lawyer and activist Angela Glover Blackwell shows in her study "The Curb-Cut Effect" that there are times when steps initially taken to aid one population—like people with disabilities— are ultimately good for all. As she recounts, in the early 1970s, pedestrian curb cuts were unheard-of in American cities. A group of wheelchair activists in Berkeley, California, frustrated about the difficulty of wheeling around their city, began pouring concrete for makeshift ramps that would ease getting on and off sidewalks.

At first, the activists were threatened with arrest, but before long the first official curb cut was made and many cities followed, as they realized what now seems obvious: The curb cuts weren't useful only for wheelchair users. Parents with strollers, workers with handcarts and travelers with luggage all benefited. This action helped people with disabilities integrate further into economic and cultural life. When I go to work, or pick up my children from school, those curb cuts help me get there.

I owe a debt to those activists, and to others whose actions helped move us toward the passage of the Americans With Disabilities Act in 1990. Now it is my turn to speak up, thank my fellow New Yorkers for their underrated kindness, and ask the transit authority to commit to follow their lead and work for all of us.

A Symbol for "Nobody" That's Really for Everybody

ELIZABETH GUFFEY

I WAS 12 YEARS OLD WHEN I FIRST ENCOUNTERED THE BLUE WHEELCHAIR symbol. I still remember sitting in our family car on that hot Southern California afternoon in 1975 as my mother pulled into the department store parking lot. Something was wrong. The cars were all parked in the wrong places. Then, as we drove near the store's front door, we saw a new set of neatly painted blue and white lines on the pavement, and a little wheelchair symbol stenciled on each space. The rest of the parking lot was filled, but these spaces were all conspicuously empty.

I especially remember the comments that came after the new spaces arrived. "It's such a shame," our neighbor told my mother one day. "It used to be if you arrived early enough you could count on getting a parking space in front of the store. Now nobody can use them." Later I wondered, who is "nobody"?

I was born with cerebral palsy. At that point I had never used a wheelchair, but as soon as I saw that figure, I knew instinctively that it was a friend and an ally. Whatever my neighbor or other people said, the little figure was whispering a message of inclusion directly to me.

To this day, I have a complicated relationship with wheelchairs. I did not use one at all until my 40s, when I first visited the New York Maker Faire in Queens, N.Y., and my wheelchair use remains peripatetic. Even so, I've long recognized this symbol as a kind of lifeline that allows me to participate in and contribute to larger society. Like many disabled people, I was born with a body that allows partial mobility. As a child, I used heavy braces and special orthotic shoes, and I've always found it challenging to merely move across a room. I fall frequently, and my injuries have included concussions, broken teeth and sprained limbs. Despite these setbacks, the symbol has guided me through places, and pointed out spaces that are safe.

In August 2018, the "wheelchair symbol," formally known as the International Symbol of Access, turned 50. It's an occasion worth celebrating.

The original symbol was conceived by Susanne Koefoed, a Danish design student during the turbulent summer of 1968—a year now remembered for social upheavals like the resistance in Prague, the strikes in Paris and the raised fists of black American athletes at the Mexico City Olympics. In the student-led design workshop in Stockholm that she was attending, Koefoed planted the seed for another sort of revolution when she came up with an idea for common signage to guide disabled people to accessible facilities. She drew a schematic wheelchair.

The icon spent a brief childhood in Sweden in the months after this workshop, where it could be seen around traffic intersections in Stockholm's center and at the city's new international airport. That same year, the symbol was adopted by the well-connected nonprofit organization Rehabilitation International. Global in reach, and with deep pockets, Rehabilitation International hoped to promote the symbol through its many media and political connections. The effort stalled, however, until officials made a simple modification—they placed a circle on top of the wheelchair's back, transforming it into an image of a *person* sitting in a wheelchair.

The symbol really took off in 1974, when the United Nations approved it as a key component of barrier-free design. Officially rendered in the now-familiar blue and white, the international convention for roadside amenities, the little icon became a familiar sight in parking lots, restrooms, ramps and other public places across the globe. In 1990, when President George H. W. Bush signed the Americans With Disabilities Act into law, the "wheelchair symbol" came to legally identify a host of standardized accommodations for disabled people. By this time, it was one of the most recognized symbols in the world. In the United States, it is now accepted as legal signage and can be found on road signs, disabled parking tags and other official documents across the 50 states.

In recent years, a number of designers have reimagined the wheelchair symbol. In 2011, Sara Hendren and Brian Glenney redesigned the symbol as part of their Accessible Icon Project in a way that reflects the wider public understanding of members of the disabled community as people who play dynamic, active roles in public life. Their design pushes the figure out of its familiar sedentary stance. It depicts a wheelchair user leaning purposefully, even forcefully forward, setting it all in motion, as though racing through traffic or over a finish line. This newer symbol is now legally accepted in New York and Connecticut as a replacement for the older icon.

It's been years since I first heard my neighbor openly complain about the wheelchair symbol, or the accommodations it is meant to provide. Today, I recognize that even then, the little figure was moonlighting. Yes, its official job remains to identify facilities and guide disabled people to ramps, automated doors or larger toilet stalls. But it also reminds us that access to buses and trains, entry to stores and classrooms, and the enjoyment of parks and pools is a legal right shared by everyone—disabled or not. And it reminds us of our fundamental obligation to support one another and to continue building the barrier-free society that we know we can build.

We can also happily note that my neighbor was wrong: The wheelchair symbol is not a design for nobody. It actually belongs to all of us.

Feeling My Way Into Blindness

EDWARD HOAGLAND

BLINDNESS IS ENVELOPING. IT'S BEYOND BELIEF TO STEP OUTSIDE AND see so little, just a milky haze. Indoors, a smothering dark. It means that you can't shed a mood of loneliness with a brisk walk down the street because you might trip, fall and break something. Nor will you see a passing friend, the sight of whom could be as cheery as an actual conversation. Sights, like sounds, randomly evoke a surge of memories ordinarily inaccessible that lighten and brighten the day. "Who are you?" I may already have asked 10 people who have spoken to me. Their body language as well as their smiles are lost to me. Human nature is striped with ambiguities, and you need to see them, but like a prisoner, I am hooded.

I lost my sight once before, to cataracts, a quarter-century ago, but it was restored miraculously by surgery. It then went seriously bad again, until, reaching 80, I needed a cane. Tap, tap. Ambulatory vision is the technical term.

Everything becomes impromptu, hour by hour improvised. Pouring coffee so it doesn't spill, feeling for the john so you won't pee on the floor, calling information for a phone number because you can't read the computer, or the book. Eating takes considerable time since you can't see your food. Feeling for the scrambled eggs with your fingers, you fret about whether you appear disgusting. Shopping for necessities requires help. So does traveling on a bus.

The kindness of strangers is proverbial—a woman leads me through the bustle of an airport toward the taxi stand, a waitress hands me back a $50 bill I mistook for a 20. Blindness is factually a handicap, yet an empathetic one, because other people can so easily imagine themselves suffering from it, sometimes even experiencing a rehearsal for it when stumbling through a darkened house at night. I remember how in school we teased students with Coke-bottle glasses, but didn't laugh at blind folk whose black glasses signified that they couldn't see at all.

I know about handicaps harder to cotton to, having stuttered terribly for decades, my face like a gargoyle's, my mouth flabbering uncontrollably. Blindness is old hat. In Africa you still see sightless souls led about by children gripping the other end of a stick. Blindness in its helplessness reassures the rest of us that that oddball is not an eyesore or a loose cannon. Being blind is omission, not commission; and you'd better learn how to fall. Paratrooper or tumbler training would be useful. A tumbler can tip sideways as he lands so his hip and shoulder absorb the blow.

The ears need schooling as a locator. I search for the bathroom at night, guided by a ticking clock whose location I recognize. As you go blind, exasperating incongruities arise, but also the convenience of this new excuse for shedding social obligations not desired. And you can give your car away.

Hearing snatches of conversation from invisible voices, everything becomes eavesdropping. Have I seen my last movie? Is the vision gone from television? But I can still see daylight and bipedal forms, tree crowns and running water, swirling, seething leaves against the sky-blue heavens, which remind me of 80 years of previous gazing on several continents. Eternal instants on Telegraph Hill, Beacon Hill, or Venice and Kampala.

Splendiferous mountain vistas of greensward and cliffs scaffold my dreams, drawn from memories of sheep pastures in Sicily and Greece, rich with textured sedges or tinted canyons, then bombastic skyscrapers, or Matisse's Chapel. So it's flabbergastingly impoverishing to wake up in the morning. Faces are no longer seamed, nor are raindrops stippled on the windowpane, cats high-tailed in a turf war, postage stamps vividly illustrative. I forget my condition and grope for my glasses, wherever they are, as if they could solve the emergency. Blindness *is* an emergency; the window shades are drawn, and one deals with it in myriad ways.

Instinctively I reach out to touch everyone I talk with, heightening the moment of contact. Shoulders I go for, as gender-neutral, companionable territory, but most folks don't want to chat for long with anyone whose deficits are front and center. There's sympathy fatigue, though allowances must be made, an elbow gripped, and perhaps the menu read aloud in a restaurant. Poor guy; be considerate; tell him what the headlines were in the paper today, but if he's not Helen Keller, let the next person take a turn at being nice.

You get somebody to scan your mail for you outside the post office, and supervise paying a bill in the return envelope, maybe even writing the check for you to sign. Improvising keeps one alive, and at the beach you can hear the surf thump if not exult in the spindrift's curl. The tide tugs your feet. At 4:30 in midsummer you hear the birds' morning chorus, nature primeval and ascendant. You dig when you're blind, fingering for roots, then for what the roots are connected to. Curiosity does tip into tediousness, though, when there's no new material.

Blindness as a metaphor is not flattering. Blind drunk, a parent blind to the misery of her children, a politician blind to the needs of his constituents. When blind you can neither read text nor frowns, but if somebody starts talking to you and you can't see them, hang loose till you figure it out. Equilibrium is the key.

Eyedrops of several descriptions and optical devices accumulate as each is superseded by another. You used different hand lenses for different phases of magnification. Since a book or film is not in the cards, blindly groping for succor in your boredom can be a danger. That comfy stranger on the bench may be Mr. Ponzi. Discipline is required. In all your parts, do you still enjoy being alive? Crossing your legs and twitching an ankle, savoring cherry tomatoes, then sweet corn and lobster.

Nights can turn bright if the world mysteriously whitens, as though one's optic nerves were rebelling. It's odd when one part of the body dies but the rest does not. In blindness we don't cast off our eyes, but continue to consult them in thwarted ways, much as amputees feel their lost parts almost function.

Feeling a chill wind, I'll look at the sky for a forecast, but triangulate the slanting breezes for the message I can't see. I smell the rain before it comes, and the sun speaks to my skin like a finger stroking. As, in my view, joy in people may be analogous to photosynthesis in plants, this is quite logical. But wet days can be delicious also, a cool drink for dry skin, restful in its implications; good weather has its pressures. Less is expected of a rainy day; you can hole up a bit with yourself.

Like Plato's Cave, your brain consists of memories flickering on a wall. The phenomenalities of sight are now memories, but my sixth sense has helped. Call it intuition; and I've never felt despair, any more than when I was a kid who couldn't talk. Blindness resembles a stretched-out stroke. Functions wither as your walking slows. Muscles atrophy and sensibilities, too. You can't size up a new visage, yet the grottoes in your head have more to plumb if your sight was lost midlife or later. You can go caving.

Where are my eyes, I suddenly think, as if I'd left behind my coat. Landscapes become impressionistic, eliding details. Abbreviation is at the core. Input is so precious—the conversations other people pause to grant you, beyond the barest niceties, describing piquant scenery you can't see. Strong sunlight is needed for a newsstand headline but muted illumination has subtler uses, and in pitch dark a blind man is at an advantage.

The personality of the street, hubbubbed with hurry, invites strolling. Slatted fences, orange lilies, SALE signs in a window. "Outta sight!" a guy exclaims. I seek a bench I know about, remembering a whole gallery of friends who have died by now. Older than Mozart, younger than Bach, they engulfed my life with love and commitment, and on a good day permeate my mind. My sexual fantasies invoke an alloy of wives and friends. But anonymity has swallowed me like Jonah's whale; I grope inside.

Sunlight beams turn the street radiant for a quarter-hour. Two of my mentors ended their lives by suicide, and I remember their dilemmas sympathetically. One jumped into the sea, the other the Mississippi, but I wonder in each case whether the sun was shining or they'd waited for a rainy day. Our elements return, in any event, to the oceans to re-form as other life.

Nature is our mother, if no longer our home. We couch-surf in rented beach houses, with green belts as habitat for other creatures that remain. How many of us have watched a possum "play possum" or a goshawk swoop after a blue jay? We feed pigeons and hummingbirds, then have done with it. Nature has become a suburb. Of course I can't see the cardinal at the feeder out the window, though tidal forces still operate. The leaves natter even if you can't see them. Your ears report their bustle, ceaseless until dormant for a span of moments. The pulse in your throat signals that in your torso all is well; it will beat till it quits. That concordance of organs lives within us like sea creatures throbbing on a coral reef, strung there as on our skeleton as long as conditions allow.

Novelty is the spice of life and salts our daily round even when we lose our sight. Your eyes don't steer you as you saunter, yet your lungs, legs, arms feel as fit as ever. For simple exercise, I hoist myself out of each chair, or bicycle in bed, though then unfortunately may pick up two completely different shoes and try to squeeze them on. My socks don't match either. But why am I not crankier? a friend asks. I'm helpless; I can't be cranky. Blindness is enforced passivity. I have become a second-class citizen, an object of concern. Crankiness won't persuade people to treat me thoughtfully. Disabled, that dry term once applied to so many others over my lifetime, now applies to me. As best I can, I'll make my peace with it.

The Athlete in Me Won't Stop

TODD BALF

"You're sort of in between, aren't you?" an old friend asked me recently.

She'd been through it all with me—my diagnosis of a rare spine cancer two years ago, the radical multistage surgery, the long rehab stint, the longer convalescence at home, and the eventual finding that I'd suffered a complication in surgery that caused a spinal cord injury and what will probably be permanent paraplegia. My sports-toned and -nurtured legs hadn't responded to rehab the way they'd been expected to because they couldn't.

What my friend was saying—and why I was nodding along—is that I don't fit in the most recognizable spinal cord injury groups. I'm not in a wheelchair anymore. I've learned to stand for long periods. My naturally dark skin tone returned once I got back outdoors. For most of my professional life I've reported and written about athletes and adventurers. I've climbed Grand Teton in Wyoming, trekked the Darien Jungle in Panama. In a photograph recently taken of me in front of my weather-beaten New England barn I look a lot like I used to. "Defiant," she said.

But I'm sure that the visit I made to her lake house a few weeks earlier was in the back of her mind. I'd joined her and a half-dozen other friends; it was my first time there since my surgery. A party barge was next to shore for easy boarding, and though I was able to edge my fanny onto the low loading deck and hoist my legs up, I couldn't get up from there. Everybody was trying to be cool and respectful but nobody knew what to do. My helplessness was striking.

I'm what's known as an "incomplete," meaning I have incomplete paralysis below the level of my spinal injury. I walk with a stock right-side cane and a discreet brace resembling a shin guard that slips into my shoe to help raise my limp left foot. When I run into people on my walking route for the first time they sometimes offer guesses as to what happened. A broken leg? A recently reconstructed hip? They're thinking a temporary condition, not paralysis.

The American Spinal Injury Association has a scale of "incompleteness" and I'm an ASIA D—meaning "more than 50 percent of the muscles spared below the level of injury are strong enough to move against gravity." At some point in recovery my muscles edged from "not useful" to "useful." In 2016, after many months of training, and a bit of adaptive tinkering, I taught myself to ride an upright pedal-assist e-bike. It has a low, step-through frame. I use clip-in pedals to help pull my "dead" left leg through the motion. Mostly I look like anyone else on a bike.

At a stop sign, however, it gets interesting. I restart with difficulty because I have to shove off skateboard-style a few times with my right leg and only once I'm coasting can I pull up my right leg with my opposing hand to place it on the pedal platform. (My right leg can't thrust upward on its own because I'm missing my psoas on that side; it was removed because the tumor was there, too.) Most times I get through an intersection without trouble. But in an early trial I stumbled and caused an embarrassing slowdown at a four-way stop. One motorist screamed something and my older brother, who was my riding partner that day, screamed back: "He's got a paralyzed left leg, OK?" It was nice of him to defend me but the motorist might've been forgiven. Paralyzed? I was on a bike.

I am close enough to the physical life I adore to touch it, close enough to feel that a brilliant physical therapist or a smart tech innovation could bring me back to it in full. But I'm still far enough away that young children stare and acquaintances offer to drive me from place to place. I can push my legs forward but I can't shake them awake for a vigorous effort. I crave that red zone feeling, the fierce power and pain that comes from big leg muscles bursting beneath you. But I can get there only in my memory.

When I was first trying to get a grip on exactly who I was now I told my physiatrist I felt like a "mishmosh." Perhaps exhausted by the prospect of a full inventory of my right and left side muscle groups and the physical "actions" they couldn't quite pull off, he simply agreed, "Yes, you're a mishmosh."

In being a part of this in-between world, still thinking I might belong to one instead of the other, there is another problem— identifying my tribe. I wish to be part of an active crowd, but it's confusing. My local fall 5-kilometer race invites runners, walkers and wheelchairs. None of those categories is quite right for me.

In a way, I identify with youthful athletes who've been tragically struck down only to rebound in some unique, indefatigable way.

But my tribe also seems to be the older, retired neighbors I see on my walks. They often encourage me. I typically get a wave and "you're doing well" (though out walking in a snowstorm one winter I did get a circumspect "you're a stubborn one, aren't you?") I have their aches and pains. I share their fears about safely getting around in a too-fast world. They look out for me.

There are a handful of psychological stages involved in coping with a disabling spinal cord injury. The final one, which the pamphlets say is the most important, is "acceptance." But I'm not accepting. I time myself on walks, use an app to chart power data in watts. I'm a little happier with myself when I set a personal record than when I don't. I think and behave like the athlete I was. I can't stop. My friends are comforted by this crazy behavior. It is in my nature, evidence that I haven't changed. I'm relentless. My eyes are on the prize.

Out on my own I can almost forget my disability. The numbness I get in my legs on walks is familiar enough now that it's almost like a weekend warrior's baggage—there, but in the background, like when the ache in a hoops player's arthritic knees vanishes at tip-off. But then, at a summer wedding on the edge of a frenetic dance floor, my differences are exposed again. I am new to this. I suspect this "them" and "us" dynamic is well known to the disability community. I'm sure I'd find shared comfort there. But I'm in limbo. To pull closer to that world feels like giving up on the other.

I am told that in some cases Mother Nature smiles upon a person with an injury like mine. I often imagine nerves lengthening and muscles awakening as I plant my legs extra purposefully on my walks, thinking in my uninformed way that mental power or an act of will might spur something I cannot know or see. And yet the window is likely closing on natural nerve regeneration. Nerve repair ordinarily happens in the first year. It's been two.

I am tempted to pursue my recovery as far as medical science will take me. I hate shutting the door on the possible. My legs made me. They defined me, carrying me for as long as I can remember across wild places, up steep, punishing trails. I'm looking at my legs now. They're beneath me. But they're not.

The Dawn of the "Tryborg"

JILLIAN WEISE

THE EXISTENCE OF "THE TRYBORG," AS A CATEGORY OF PERSON, IS SO obvious that once I point it out, you will immediately recognize a dozen tryborgs you know or whose work you have read. It is possible you are a tryborg.

The company that makes my leg calls it a C-Leg, a cruel name, since it is vulnerable to salt water and cannot go anywhere near the sea. I've been wearing prosthetic legs for over 30 years. In the last decade, I've been wearing a leg with a computerized knee. The knee weighs 2.8 pounds and lasts 40 to 45 hours on a charge. I vacuum seal into my leg, so the boundary where I end and computer begins is imperceptible to me.

Our best-known cyborgs have long been fictional (think Lee Majors as "The Six Million Dollar Man"), but today we are real. Most cyborgs are disabled people who interface with technology. We depend on a computer for some major bodily function. The tryborg—a word I invented—is a nondisabled person who has no fundamental interface. The tryborg is a counterfeit cyborg. The tryborg tries to integrate with technology through the latest product or innovation. Tryborgs were the first to wear Google Glass. Today they wait in line for Snapchat Spectacles. The tryborg adopts the pose of a cyborg. But no matter how hard they try, the tryborg remains a pretender.

The tryborg may be an early adopter, a pro gamer, a TED Talker, a content creator or a follower. The tryborg may be an expert who writes about cyborgs for screenplays, lab reports or academic journals. The tryborg may just be a guy named Bob who works in I.T. and collects Real Dolls. Whatever the case: Tryborgs can only imagine what life is like for us.

The tryborg is always distanced by metaphor, guesswork and desire. When my leg suddenly beeps and buzzes and goes into "dead mode"—the knee stiffens; I walk like a penguin—the tryborg is alive without batteries. When I sound like a bomb in a liquor store, the tryborg hurries on, nonelectronic.

Tryborgs want to be cyborgs. This is why they go to bed with Fitbit, brag about gigabit and buy kit with Bitcoin. They have an affinity for the it or the Id. But even when they find a mate by swiping right, and then tell that mate how many steps they walked since Sunday, still they are not cyborgs. To mistake them for cyborgs is to confuse the figurative with the literal.

If you are thinking, No, no, no, cyborgs do not exist, they are theoretical creatures, then you are likely a tryborg.

Tryborgs rely on the nonexistence of actual cyborgs for their bread and butter. If cyborgs exist, how will the tryborg remain relevant? Wouldn't we just ask the cyborg for her opinion? The opinions of cyborgs are conspicuously absent from the expert panels, the tech leadership conferences and the advisory boards. The erasure is not news to us. We have been deleted for centuries, and in the movies, you will often see us go on a long, fruitful journey, only to delete ourselves in the end.

But anyone with a hard drive can tell you: Even when you delete something, it is not really gone. So it is with us cyborgs. We remain in the periphery, un-scrubbed and un-snuffed out.

Maybe tryborgs imagine that the theorist Donna Haraway's "A Cyborg Manifesto" is right. The manifesto reads: "In short, we are cyborgs. The cyborg is our ontology; it gives us our politics." But Haraway is a tryborg: She's not disabled; she has no interface; she uses the term as a metaphor. The strategic move where one group says, "I shall speak for them because they do not exist / do not live here / do not have thoughts" is common of the tryborg. When they are not speaking for us, they may take a detour into animal studies, a field where they can rest assured that their subjects remain silent.

Other tryborgs of note include Jaron Lanier ("You Are Not a Gadget"—well, what if I am?), Michio Kaku ("Physics of the Future") and Ray Kurzweil ("The Age of Intelligent Machines"). Tryborgs need not be famous, though they often try to sell us things: vodka, car accidents or exoskeletons. Tryborgs are often company men, selling us the future, which they imagine will be populated first by male cyborgs. This is why so many cyborg headlines concern men and their inventions: the Lovetron 9000, a vibrating penis; "Captain Cyborg," who wears an ultrasonic baseball cap so he can be just like the blind.

I know it will take time, but things will change. For a while, all the experts on African-Americans were white. All the experts on lesbians were Richard von Krafft-Ebing. All the experts on cyborgs were noninterfaced humans.

Please do not be sad. It should bring us great relief to know who we are. The Delphic oracle declares it: Know thyself. It is not my fault if we have been taking liberties with metaphor, clicking along, declaring ourselves this, when really we are that. As the Stanford professor Franco Moretti once said, "Somehow digital humanities has managed to secure for itself this endless infancy, in which it is always a future promise." Cyborgs are tired of being your babies.

"You just have a chip on your shoulder," says the tryborg, smiling down from Google headquarters (the futurist factory) in Mountain View, California.

No, I have a chip in my knee. But I accept your invitation. I am in talks with your futurists, although in poetry, the code I prefer.

I will be your cyborg laureate.

For our first order of business: Will you please, kind sirs, create computerized parts for women? If you can give a man goat legs and a second stomach to chew cud, then surely you can give a woman legs. All the computerized parts are made in the image of men. You object: "What about Heather Mills and Aimee Mullins?" Yes, they can afford designer legs. Aimee Mullins owns 12 pairs of legs. The plebeian cyborg owns one.

Take my C-Leg. It gives me the muscular calf of a man-cyclist. I have a ruler, and the company name, on my shin. I can choose between the colors Volcano Shadow or Desert Pearl, which is to say, gray or brownish-gray. I cannot choose a female option because there are none. I have no complaint about androgyny. But I'm just a regular femme who likes to show her legs. Yes, I have come this far, to beg that you make a leg look like a woman's leg.

Second, why place the outlet on my calf? How many women do you know who want their outlets exposed? To plug myself in, I must decide between uncomfortable positions. Either I remove my leg and kneel beside it as if in prayer to the tryborg creation. Or I leave my leg on and plug in by making a certain kind of pose absent from all the yoga charts. Is it tree? Is it boat?

Finally, I do not like the way I must maintain a specific weight, not to exceed 110 pounds, if I want to walk on two legs. I would like to get fatter like the rest of you. This computerized leg corsets me.

My own expert, the salesman from the leg company, asked me to name my leg for the app. The app is called "Cockpit" because of course it is. I can calibrate for skiing, golfing or cycling. Those are, apparently, the only sports I wish to pursue. The salesman had a buzz cut, shiny shoes and efficiency. He could've been a cyborg, if someone had been there to accidentally jitter his heart or remove his arm.

"Call me Foxy," I said.

Flying While Blind

GEORGINA KLEEGE

"BUT WHAT ABOUT ME?"

Those words were spoken by a man sitting next to me on an airplane. I was in the aisle seat and he was in the center. He was speaking to the flight attendant who was delivering the preflight safety briefing. Usually, I will get a private briefing during the preboarding process for people with disabilities. But this time, a flight attendant didn't get to me until the plane was fully boarded.

In the language of the boarding announcement, I am "someone who needs a little extra time going down the Jetway." This is not entirely true. I am blind, but I am a fast walker, particularly in the unobstructed space of Jetways and airplanes where there are rarely obstacles or intersections to make a wrong turn. I can lift my own suitcase into the overhead bin. I am very tall, making the lift and twist easier, and I know how to pack light. Usually, all I need is help finding my seat, though I can often accomplish this simply by counting.

Sometimes the flight attendants will realize I am an experienced traveler and abbreviate the briefing. Yes, I know how to buckle my seatbelt and that the nearest exit might be behind me. Sometimes they have a Braille version of the safety information card. This makes for interesting reading, because in describing the position to take in case of a crash landing, there's greater precision than in the image alone. Once in a while, they even let me handle the oxygen mask and life jacket, which allows me to retain a tactile memory of those objects that I hope will come back to me should the need arise.

While all this is going on I strive to reassure the attendant that I won't be any extra work for her during the flight. I am not only an experienced traveler, I am an experienced blind person, too. I know how to find my way to the lavatory. In the unlikely event that food is served, I know how to feed myself.

Part of the standard safety briefing is to tell me that in case of emergency, I should stay where I am and wait for a member of the crew to come back and rescue me. It does not take much imagination to predict that in the chaos of some disaster, this is unlikely to happen. How is the flight attendant going to get to me if the aisle is clogged with my fellow passengers rushing toward the exit?

The man in the seat next to me, idly eavesdropping as she got to this part of her spiel, piped up, "But what about me?" His tone was aggrieved, perhaps a little anxious. He went on to point out that if I remained seated in the event of this hypothetical emergency, he would have to climb over me, and those few extra seconds might be the difference between life and death.

I had to think fast. The two of them were talking about and around me, and I was vanishing from the conversation. This is a familiar experience for many disabled people, and it can be risky to remain silent. It seemed urgent to reshape the image of myself as a barrier and burden, so I said, "If the lights go out, or there's smoke and no visibility, I can lead the way."

I felt a bit guilty using this ploy, because I was ascribing value to myself that other passengers, particularly other disabled passengers, could not claim. I was thinking of a man who preboarded with me, now sitting a couple of rows ahead. He was in a wheelchair in the Jetway but walked onto the plane on his own. He explained to me somewhat sheepishly, that he was "just a little shaky on my pins." I suspect he worried that I, a legitimate disabled person, would denounce him as an impostor.

Like many people I meet preboarding airplanes or waiting in

what I think of as the disability holding pens, where we wait for assistants to move us around, he did not consider himself to be a person with a disability in his everyday life. I wanted to tell him that the problem was not his shaky pins; the problem was that airports are disabling spaces. The vast distances of long concourses can be daunting. Signage is often hard to decipher even for people with average vision. Announcements compete with each other in a garbled sonic mess.

When people avail themselves of disability services at airports, riding wheelchairs and golf carts and boarding before everyone else, we also find ourselves subject to policies about emergency protocols, such as the requirement to remain in our seats and wait for help.

Still thinking fast, I resisted the urge to list my academic and professional accomplishments as proof that I am a clear thinker, accustomed to directing others, good in a crisis. Fortunately, my fellow passenger only needed to consider for a second. "Yeah," he said, "she can get around in the dark. She could lead me to safety."

I couldn't tell for sure, but I assessed that the man was young to middle-aged and physically fit. When I stood up to let him in the seat I observed that he was above average in height. He had flipped his suitcase into the overhead bin with ease. His broad shoulders extended beyond the width of his seat. I considered pointing out that in the hypothetical disaster, as I led him to the exit, we could also assist Mr. Shaky-on-my-pins. For all we knew, he might be a physician, or a former Boy Scout, ready to administer first aid. Who knew what valuable skills he might have in a disaster? Between the two of us, surely my seatmate and I could get him out as well.

The flight attendant was a bit flummoxed. My fellow passenger was displaying a kind of defiance in his solidarity with me. Perhaps this is why they usually conduct these briefings before the nondisabled people board. She decided not to argue with us, and that was the end of it.

As we taxied to take off, I became aware that my seatmate was gripping the armrest between us. I could feel the tension in his elbow pressing against my arm. I realized that I had misjudged him. His seeming physical fitness had distracted me from the possibility that he might be a fearful flyer. I wanted to say something reassuring, but I sensed that my presence and the disastrous scenario it had compelled him to imagine had triggered his anxiety. So I resorted to the tried-and-true small talk of travelers: Was this trip business or pleasure? Was he leaving home or on his way back? I am an experienced traveler; I know how people talk. Soon enough, he released his grip on the armrest, the wheels left the tarmac and we were on our way.

V

COPING

My Life With Paralysis, It's a Workout

VALERIE PIRO

THE ALARM GOES OFF AT 4:30 A.M. GROGGY, I TURN ON THE LAMP ON my night stand and try to sit up. I put my right hand on the wall next to my bed to steady myself, and push my left into the bed. Right away, my abs and back seize up and my legs spasm and kick out straight, forcing me back down onto the bed. Clearly my body thinks it is too early to get up, but I don't have time to argue with it. I have to get physical therapy out of the way so I can be on time for my medieval history class.

After I sit up, I place my hands under my right knee and clasp them together as I bring my knee up and closer to my chest. I reach out to my right foot and cross its heel over my left thigh so that I can plant my heel on the bed. I hug my right leg against my torso and chest and feel a stretch in my lower back and butt. I repeat this on my other side and then proceed to stretch each ankle.

Paralysis requires maintenance.

I then hop toward the foot of my bed, where my commode chair sits. I set both feet on the footrests as best I can, grab the armrest on the far side of the chair with my left hand, and, using my right hand to drive down into my bed, lift myself onto the commode wheelchair, and wheel to the bathroom.

I emerge at 5:35 a.m. I transfer now into a wheelchair whose dimensions are friendly toward my Functional Electrical Stimulation (F.E.S.) cycle—something like a gym exercise bike, without the seat. I pull some milk out of the mini-fridge and pour it over a bowl of cereal. I eat while checking and answering email. At 6:30 it's time to start cycling. I put two small rectangular electrodes on my left shin muscles, and then two on my right, connect them to the cycle, then strap in my legs and feet. Then two more electrodes then two more, and so on, until most of my lower body is tapped and wired. After I turn on the tablet that's attached to the cycle, I choose from one of several preset programs to start my workout. Within a couple of minutes, electrical shocks are pulsing into my legs, causing them to contract into pedaling. Imagine pedaling a bicycle uphill for an hour; this is my workout.

Still, I'm groggy. I spend the hour feeling various muscles contract, occasionally nodding off and jerking back awake, and thinking about paper topics for my three history classes, a Latin translation I need ready by the next day and an email I need to send an adviser, and wondering if I should keep my laptop next to my cycle for the next workout so I can pedal and binge watch "30 Rock."

OK, almost there.

At 8 I take my electrodes off, bag them and transfer back into my bathroom wheelchair and wheel to my shower. By 9, I am mostly dressed. I transfer to a third wheelchair, a power-assist whose batteries had been charging overnight. I have 30 minutes to blow-dry my hair, make sure my bag is packed, apply enough makeup to cover my acne, and put on my sneakers and jacket, before heading to the shuttle that will take me to my college's main campus.

By 9:45, I'm outside my Making the Middle Ages class. I wave slowly at a classmate across the hall.

"Hey, how are you?" she asks, "You look tired."

"No, that's just my face," I say, and laugh a little. If you've read this far, you'll understand why I didn't go into more detail just then. My mornings are complicated.

I have never felt comfortable discussing my physical therapy regimen with other students, particularly if I do not know them well. I learned in high school that if I discussed my disability, physical therapy or any inevitable difficulties that came with the mobility-impaired life, that no one wanted to continue the conversation.

My high school track teammates who visited me in the hospital after my spinal cord injury met my stories with awkward silence when I returned to finish my senior year. Some of the captains discouraged me from speaking with new team members. I was a reminder of the van we were in that rolled down a highway median (I was injured the most seriously). They felt uncomfortable looking at me. And when I got into Harvard, they insinuated that my acceptance was a result of affirmative action. More than one classmate told me, in words that varied only slightly, that I was lucky to have a "perfect personal essay topic." (I attended Stuyvesant in New York City, where students have an unhealthy obsession with getting into elite colleges and any life obstacle was considered an edge for getting into an Ivy League school.) Halfway through senior year, my friends became nothing more than signatures on the large get well card they gave me the year before.

My high school teammates' discomfort wormed its way into how I talked about my disability during my four years of college. I wanted to keep my college friends, and silence on certain topics seemed the best option. Similarly, I wanted my professors to know that I took my work seriously, and so I would go to class even when my blood pressure was low enough that I was close to fainting, or when my body temperature had dropped to the point where I could not stop visibly shivering in class. When my disability made it difficult to work, it was the last thing I would use to explain an absence from class.

I was concerned that my situation would immediately fall into a stereotyped narrative—either disability as tragedy or disability as my personal hurdle I sought to overcome as I desperately worked to rejoin the able-bodied. I feared that my disability could not exist as it was.

To avoid labels, I played down any improvements I made in physical therapy, choosing to tell my friends about how my arms were jacked instead of how my hip flexors were finally showing trace movement. There was another angle: If I mentioned improvement, it implied that I hated my disabled body and wished for what the able-bodied perceive as normal. If I mentioned that I exercised my legs to avoid atrophy so that I may be able to benefit if there was ever a cure for paralysis, I worried over betraying the disability rights cause.

We, the disabled, encourage one another to demand that society accept us for who we are, and not change our routines to accommodate how the general public feels we should look. But I want to stay healthy, and I want to keep my body ready for the future. I believe strongly that everything should have been made accessible yesterday, but I also would choose an abled version of myself over my current self any day—it's easier and more time-efficient to manage. Does spending so much time maintaining my body make me an inspiration, or a disability rights failure? Can I choose a lifestyle that won't be judged?

Perhaps not. And so I've taken on a small but meaningful act of resistance, by changing the way I talk about the life I now lead. I've sought to explain my regimen to others as health maintenance, which is an accurate, although thoroughly unsexy, description. My F.E.S. cycle workouts and standing frame (a machine that is exactly what it sounds like) sessions keep my muscles and bone density intact, my circulation going, and my health at a level such that I am less likely to require hospitalization.

I don't want to come off as angry, hopeless or inspirational, because my life may end up defined by one of those adjectives if I provide the slightest description of my day. But let me, just for now, take control of my story and tell you that I have a disability, and it takes time and effort to both maintain my health and live my life.

My $1,000 Anxiety Attack

JoANNA NOVAK

I HOIST MY CARRY-ON INTO OVERHEAD STORAGE, HOPING I WON'T DROP A suitcase packed with an espresso machine on the man who offered to help. "I think I've got this," I say, unsure of my volume. The new noise-canceling headphones make talking awkward, but like sunglasses, they're vital to my survival. Middle seat, seventh row, I quadruple-check: The Xanax is in my purse. This is my attempt to be fine.

I've had anxiety attacks for 20 years. They started when I was 13, a fun perk of anorexia, buy one get one free. Anorexia became bulimia and the attacks persisted, rattling like odd pennies in a piggy bank until a few years ago a new therapist compounded my diagnosis: eating disorder (not otherwise specified) *with* comorbid dysthymia and generalized anxiety disorder.

In-flight panic, though, is new-new. Lately, every tilt of the ailerons, every whiff of fuel, will cause me to periscope in my seat, searching the flight attendants' eyes for concern. Every human with two cellphones will make me think: terrorist? Even as the aircraft reaches cruising altitude, my anxiety will escalate. I'll dry-heave in the lavatory, splashing my face with nonpotable water. It's not until the plane lands that I'll take an unobstructed breath.

The woman in the seventh-row window seat studies a folio. Beside her I fuss, trying to make my personal space impervious to fear, opening my purse, ponytailing my hair, wedging a book in the seat back, finding my phone, tapping the beaming infant icon of Noobie Soothie, the white-noise app I bought when I got the headphones.

But I'm too nervous to open the Xanax.

Lots of people take it, my therapist told me. I paid for the prescription, the headphones, the Noobie Soothie, but I wasn't happy. I deciphered the receipts with a self-deprecating magic decoder ring: You're getting worse. You can't strong-arm yourself into neurotypicality. Some days, you don't even like to buy *food.* Maybe flying with anxiety is too much for you.

You don't need Xanax, I tell myself in Row 7. Your armaments against anxiety are strong enough. I stow my purse and close my eyes behind my sunglasses. Static crashes in my headphones, and for a moment, my mind hushes.

"Ladies and gentleman, we're a completely full flight," the attendant says.

I blink. Someone has unwrapped something tuna. The aisle is choked with people frowning at the prospects for their baggage. My pulse migrates from my chest to my throat. The last occupant of the seventh row arrives.

The man who takes the aisle seat next to me looks about my age. He's tall, walleyed and bushy browed. Cologne, khakis. He does human things: clicks his seatbelt, reaches into a pocket, places a phone on the armrest between us. Then, contorting, he goes to another pocket and sets another phone facedown on his thigh.

Two phones. It's clear: We're doomed.

Here's what happens in my pre-takeoff anxiety attack: The man toggles between devices, glancing—deviously, I decide. My heart batters that hush from two minutes ago. I throw side-eye behind my sunglasses. I read my neighbor's texts. They're in an app with orange bubbles, in an alphabet I don't recognize. I twist and turn in my seat, giraffe my neck, telekinetically press the "call flight attendant" button, gulp enough air to inflate a balloon, cloud my sunglasses with tears, sweat through my dress, think: This is it, the plane will be hijacked, I'll die, and my fear that flying in an airplane is reckless and dumb will be confirmed.

"Cabin doors closed for departure."

I emit a low, nauseated-animal noise, like a cow going, "Oh, god."

The two-phoned man turns and in a soft voice asks, "Are you OK?"

I shake my head and stumble toward the cockpit, where a flight attendant brews coffee. I'm panting. That same cow groan happens again.

"I'm having an anxiety attack," I tell her. "There's a man with two phones." "What's going on, honey? Deeeeeeeep breaths." My mouth trembles. My eyes dart. My heart somersaults into my brain. "I have to get off the plane," I say.

The flight attendant asks if I have luggage and I follow her to the seventh row. I struggle to pull down my carry-on and the man with two phones asks if he can help.

"Sure." I am too shocked at what I've done to look at him; everyone on the plane is too shocked at what I'm doing to stop looking at me.

I drag my bag up the jet bridge and stand at the empty gate, winded. Stranded. And headphones blasting white noise at my neck. Also, I'm broke.

When my bulimia was at its worst, I used to see the ice cream I'd purged in the kitchen sink and think of all the money I'd vomited over the years. I realize now that it can cost just as much to "manage" a mental illness, like I do, as it does to treat it medically. In 2016, Health Affairs reported mental disorders cost the United States more than any other medical condition: in 2013, $203 billion. That $203 billion accounts for psychologists, psychiatrists, inpatient and outpatient treatment, hypnosis, medication, but what about the staggering expenses the figure could never include, the private hacks people like me make to MacGyver life? Headphones. Noobie Soothie. One-thousand-dollar replacement tickets.

That's what it comes down to, in the end. I'm traveling across the country: I can't become the grown-up Eloise of the airport hotel. No bus, train or rental car solves the cost-risk-time equation better than a plane. When anxiety is related to death (mine is), of course it's about life, which means it's obsessed with choice, and therefore fixated on money. But being stingy with self-care (when you can afford it) is a dangerous habit to cultivate. It's gambling with karma: Not everyone will be able to afford these hacks.

Twenty minutes later, I head to the ticketing counter, buy two new tickets, and by the time I go through security again, I'm not just telling myself to be brave, I'm remembering that I'm grateful. Grateful there are more flights. Grateful to have a credit card and a steady job so I can pay it off. Grateful to be healthy enough to be *trying* to keep anxiety from ruling my life.

I am even grateful when my carry-on is inspected, again. I ask for a female TSA agent—my bag is an explosion of loose tampons— and we go to a glassed-in privacy room. The agent hefts my bag onto the table and I apologize for its weight. The espresso machine.

She swabs the machine with a blue-gloved finger. "This is my favorite," she says. "Expensive, but, yah know, worth it."

I'm cleared and together we struggle with the zipper. "It's possible," I say. "Another agent and I did it a couple hours ago."

The agent is sympathetic when I explain how I've already gone through security. I tell her everything, about the man, the phones, the second set of tickets, the Xanax I didn't take. She doesn't back away or hurry me along. She pauses, talking to me like a big sister.

"You have to take Xanax," she says. "I do. Even half before shift. Lotta crazy people out there. Take a Xanax and get some wine. You gotta do that."

I've been warned about mixing Xanax and alcohol. It's a no-no. But I thank her anyway. And I think about how, back in eighth grade, when I was trying to recover from anorexia, I kept quarters in my pencil case. I told friends it was my "assertiveness fund." It was money for a snack or if I ever worked up the nerve to have a regular Coke. I still haven't had a regular Coke, but when I board my next plane, I pop a pill. I shake a coin from the piggy bank.

When Life Gave Me Lemons, I Had a Panic Attack

GILA LYONS

O NE AFTERNOON SEVERAL MONTHS AGO, A FRIEND INVITED ME TO come to her house to pick from her tree brimming with Meyer lemons, my favorite. It was the magical week in Oakland, California, when lemons are ripe and fat.

This decision was not as simple as it might seem. My panic disorder made it a daunting one.

Come on, I thought, *I should be able to drive eight minutes for free fruit.* I weighed both sides—go and experience excruciating fear and physical discomfort, or stay home and let yet another activity be slashed from my repertoire. I asked a friend to come with me; she couldn't. My boyfriend was away. I could have waited another day or until later that night when more friends were home. But I wanted them, now, and I wanted my life back.

I could no longer teach, or stay home alone. I could no longer drive, sleep, shop, shower, wait in any kind of line, eat at a restaurant, or sometimes eat anything at all. I couldn't make it to therapy anymore, or sometimes even to the kitchen for a glass of water. Everyday activities went through an exhaustive cost-benefit analysis. Was it worth the panic attack I'd endure to return the book to the library? After too many panic attacks at Trader Joe's, I stopped shopping. After too many while driving, I didn't drive. But the lemons were calling.

I sat in my car, gathering courage to turn the key. Sweat drenched the armpits of my thin T-shirt, my breathing grew shallow and short.

I turned the key and my heart sped. I started driving, and dizziness and nausea clawed at my throat, threatening to blur my vision. I quickly pulled over, gulped some water, spilling half of it down my shirt, and turned the car around. *It's not worth it*, I said aloud. *It's OK, go home.* I drove home, got in bed and didn't get up for weeks.

Panic disorder has defined and limited my life since I was a child. Some years I am powerful and capable, teaching, enjoying electrifying relationships and travel. Other years I'm utterly felled, conscribed to my bed with shards of relationships, career and my health around me.

In 2017 I wrote a profile of Haben Girma, a disability rights activist and deaf-blind lawyer. Ms. Girma is the first deaf-blind graduate of Harvard Law School, as well as the first deaf-blind person I've met who skis, surfs, ballroom dances and performs improv comedy. She has traveled extensively all over the world with the help of friends and her guide dog, Maxine.

I was amazed at all Ms. Girma is able to do with accommodations like assistive technology and interpreters. After the article was published, I disclosed to her that, while very different, I've also had to work my way around a handicap. She asked me, with utmost compassion and gentleness, if I considered myself disabled. I'd never thought of myself as such, but it was if a light had been switched on.

Because of panic, I'd been unable to attend conferences, weddings, vacations and a host of other financially gainful, career-promoting and socially enjoyable activities. But it seemed like that was just part of being me. If I'd had to pass up jobs and miss vacations because of an overtly physical condition, there would be no question I was dealing with a disability. But because mine was psychological, it seemed a personality quirk, my own sensitivities, an unfortunate trait.

In the summer of 2017 I was accepted to a prestigious fellowship that offered to fly me around the world and put me up in a hotel so that I could network with other artists, activists, educators and entrepreneurs. If I were blind, a guide dog or human aide could help guide me safely through the airport; if I were in a wheelchair, the conference would provide an attendee to help me navigate the building. But how could I make the plane, and being so far from home, accessible for my panic disorder?

Ms. Girma directed me to The Job Accommodation Network, a site that guides employees and employers to accommodate disabilities. But how can the world be made accessible to someone with 20/20 vision who can't drive because of panic attacks? Whose legs are structurally sound but keep buckling with adrenaline and fear? I had to decline.

In no way do I think navigating a mental disorder is harder than a physical disability. It's not. But physical disabilities are understood and written into law and accommodated, while mental illnesses are stigmatized, nebulous to measure and accommodate, and often seen as a fault in the person, rather than an uncontrollable physical reality.

The Americans With Disabilities Act protects those with both physical and mental disabilities by ensuring they have fair and equal access to employment, housing, transportation and governmental services. The Social Security Administration recognizes anxiety disorders, along with eight other categories of mental disorders, as conditions that qualify for disability benefits (financial and transportation assistance, assistive technology and more). The National Alliance on Mental Illness reports that roughly nine million Americans receive S.S.D.I. (financial benefits), 35.2 percent of which is because of a mental health condition.

But what is a mental illness and what is a normal emotional distress brought on by the vicissitudes of life? Consensus among the National Alliance on Mental Illness, the National Institute of Mental Health and the American Psychiatric Association points to mental illness as significant changes in thinking, feeling or behavior coupled with an inability to function in daily life in terms of self-care, maintaining jobs and relationships.

The National Alliance on Mental Illness reports that 20 percent of Americans experience a mental health disorder in any given year and that 5 percent live with a sustained and serious one. The National Comorbidity Survey Replication found that half of Americans will meet the DSM-IV criteria for a mental disorder in their lifetime. It is not, as the media likes to spin mass shootings and domestic abuse, characterized by violent behavior.

To qualify as disabled under Social Security guidelines, according to Anxiety Impairment Listing 12.06, one must have a diagnosis of anxiety disorder characterized by three or more of the following: restlessness, difficulty concentrating, irritability, muscle tension, sleep disturbance, fatigue. A person must also prove the impossibility of holding a job and a limitation in understanding, remembering or applying information; interacting with others; concentrating on, persisting in or completing tasks; or general life upkeep (paying bills, cooking, shopping, dressing, personal hygiene).

A person can also qualify if the disorder has been medically documented as "serious and persistent" for two years or longer or is manageable only because he or she is living in a therapeutic setting or is receiving ongoing medical treatment, therapy or psychosocial support that enables functioning.

According to these guidelines, I more than qualify. But I haven't applied, and I don't plan to.

My father pleads with me not to consider myself disabled or portray myself as such to employers or friends. He considers it a self-fulfilling prophecy. "If you start telling people you can't drive, then you won't force yourself to drive," he says. "You have to push against this." Because it's psychological, or at least manifests that way, it still seems to him that I can exercise control over it.

Sometimes I can fight against it. But sometimes I really can't. My fight-or-flight reaction is too strong. Anyone with a chronic illness like Lyme disease or fibromyalgia knows that you have good days, when you can afford to push yourself, and bad days, when the toll it will take to do a simple task is not worth the consequences you'll face later (exhaustion, pain, relapse).

It's such an American ideal, to feel we should be able to do whatever we set our minds to, physical or mental limitations be damned. We are taught that no matter what stands in our way, the triumphant overcome it in pursuit of a goal, picking ourselves up by our bootstraps.

To get the lemons or to call it a day? To fight for how I want my life to be or accept the limitations of my condition? American law considers me someone with a disability. I'm not sure what I consider myself.

Am I Too Embarrassed to Save My Life?

JANE EATON HAMILTON

THE RESTAURANT IS CLOSE, SHE SAYS. IT'S RIGHT HERE.
I am walking after a reading in Toronto with a fellow writer, who's leading us to a restaurant. With each step, everything in my body bursts—angina, shortness of breath, the scream of bursitis in my hip, the knowledge of sure heart failure ahead. The road she had described as flat is actually a gradual incline that might as well be Mount Everest. I need a scooter, a car.

Can I call a cab? I ask. Come on, she repeats, it's close.

Close, where? I want to ask, but it is hard to shape words while in extremis. I want to say, "I can't," yet I don't want to draw attention to my need. As I find so often when I'm out with able-bodied companions, "right here" keeps moving further away.

Among my clearest memories of the world—of London, New York, Los Angeles, Paris, Athens, Kyoto and Shanghai—are of streets and sidewalks winding away from me, asphalt gray, their rises unending and impossible. My clearest memory of Paris is of subway stations with interminable passageways to the trains and being brought to tears.

The woman knows something of my disability, and offers some help, but not enough. She slings my computer bag over her shoulder and yanks my travel bag behind. Still, even with her burden, she walks too fast for me. There are no cabs for me to flag. I struggle on but stay silent, hoping as I have for decades that this won't be the day I die.

In 1984, when I was 30, I was diagnosed with cervical cancer—carcinoma in situ. If you have to have cancer, that's the type to get. I educated myself about my disease and sailed through treatment. But my brush with mortality shattered my idea of the world and what I expected from it. Nine months later, I had a heart attack. My body had dispensed two of the major killer diseases in less than a year? No.

When I had the heart attack I went to the hospital. The doctor refused to do more than blood work because I was "the wrong age and gender for a heart attack." He gave me Tylenol with codeine for pain and sent me home. The heart attack lasted 12 more hours and caused permanent damage to my heart muscle.

When I got a diagnosis of coronary artery disease weeks later, I had to choose between open-heart surgery, which I was convinced I couldn't survive, or long-term medical treatment. I chose the latter. Along with exhaustion and worry for my kids, who were 4 and 7 years old at the time, all I felt was shame, a heavy, pressing blanket of shame.

In the years that followed, I was exhausted and sick. I had angina attacks every time I walked or otherwise exerted myself.

I began to have joint problems around 1990, but anything that wasn't life-threatening, I ignored. In 1994, I developed heart failure, which very gradually worsened until, around 2009, it went from mild to moderate, affecting most everyday activities. If I exerted myself, my ankles would swell and my lungs would fill, followed by months of cardiac asthma and coughing.

What really sent me downhill fast was the end of my 18-year marriage. My heart function worsened and I got shortness of breath from further-narrowing arteries. Several stents were implanted but failed within months, and my bouts of severe arrhythmias grew longer and more frequent.

For four months, I suffered undiagnosed unstable angina, and then I had another heart attack, resulting in more cardiac damage, for which I got yet another stent and then open-heart surgery. But even after that major procedure, heart failure, angina and arrhythmias continued unabated until I was so short of breath I had to crawl to the bathroom. Finally, doctors discovered I was suffering from atrial fibrillation (a dangerous kind of irregular heartbeat) and in December 2015, I had cardiac ablation to steady my heart rhythm, which kicked in three months later.

Still, for all that's been fixed, I've never managed to bounce back. My exhaustion is profound; I still have shortness of breath during exertion and every activity needs to be balanced against how long it will take to recover from it. I've become nearly a shut-in.

Each one of my symptoms on its own is disabling, and together they brew up an internal hurricane. But we expect disability to be visible; we require the disabled to *look* impaired. I could always pass. Around me, people were in wheelchairs, had mobility devices, used Braille and seeing-eye dogs.

I had none of that, yet I proclaimed disability? People disagreed. I was screamed at for using disabled parking, told I didn't qualify for benefits (Meals on Wheels wasn't suitable for "someone like me"), told I was lazy, denied friendships ("*my* friends show up"), accused of faking it or of having angina only when it was convenient. I'd also hear rambling nonsense telling me coronary artery disease was karma, and I was atoning for my abuses of others in a prior life. A few people opined that my illness was God's punishment for being homosexual.

But never feigning extra-incapacity was important to me. In all these years, I've never faked a symptom. That matters not a whit to anyone else (nor could I prove it), but it's a badge of personal pride to me.

Still, having coronary artery disease, an old white guy's disease, so young was humiliating. I was a feminist lesbian. We were supposed to be strong and independent. We weren't supposed to need. My disease meant I was all need.

I thought I had somehow caused my own heart disease. I did

not drink, do drugs or eat a lot of junk food, and I was not over-weight. Was it stress? Maybe I just couldn't handle life. Eventu-ally, I discovered it's very likely I have an autoimmune disease that caused systemic and continual inflammation, itself a factor in hardening arteries. This disease explains my arthritic pain in my hips and knees, the hair loss of my childhood and more symp-toms. It's late, but finally I have a logical reason for the wreckage of my physical life.

I needed any help anyone was willing to offer. I still do. But utility is not a good building block for relationships, and so I pre-tend that my need is less acute. *I can do it, I can do it, I can do it.* I knew every excuse to slow the pace. Undone shoelace (good for two, maybe even three stops); coughing and bending double in a faux flu attack (while digging for nitro); stopping dead and throw-ing up my arms in the middle of a sentence as if a self-captivating speaker; a dropped tube of lip balm, a cover for another spritz of nitro.

Every day with a disability is a bad situation from which I can't extricate myself. I'm feeble and vulnerable. If someone brandished a knife at me on the street and shouted, "Run!" I couldn't. If I went to a protest and was pepper-sprayed or detained without access to my cardiac medications, I'd promptly die. So I sit, mostly alone, on the border of life, watching others lead it.

———

There! There! I spy a restaurant, more than a block ahead. A block! So hopelessly far! I resolve to make it to those patio chairs. How to explain my horror as my friend stomps on past them, to explain my panic as eventually we come on a whole strip of restaurants yet, still, pass one, two, three? I feel my body refusing: No, no more. How to explain how flabbergasted I am when we arrive at our des-tination and there's a flight of stairs?

Am I going up? Will I finally express how physically challenged I really am? Or am I still too embarrassed to save my life?

My Paralympic Blues

EMILY RAPP BLACK

THE WOMAN TO MY LEFT WANTS TO KNOW WHAT HAPPENED TO ME. We're in a cycling studio, where for one hour we've been pedaling away, dripping sweat, with disco lights strobing across the spandex-clad instructor at the front of the class.

I recite my familiar script while struggling to unbuckle a heavy shoe. I lost my leg at 4; I wear a prosthesis; no, it wasn't cancer; yes, it goes all the way up; no, it doesn't hurt; no, I don't know that woman who was on "Dancing With the Stars," or the other lady on the other show who tap danced and was maybe married to a Beatle; and oh, how great that you had an uncle who wore a wooden leg who had a good sense of humor *in spite of all that*; yeah, bummer about that famous handsome athlete with no legs who killed his girlfriend. "Gives them a bad name," the woman says, shaking her head.

I'm used to fielding these questions, used to being lumped in as one of "them," although I find tap dancing irritating and have zero in common with a South African male double amputee professional sprinter convicted of murder. I'm so practiced at telling my story that I anticipate my cycle mate's response before I hear it. "Well, you're an inspiration! If you can do it, no excuse for me!"

My new buddy presses her hand to her heart before raising it high in the air for a sweaty fist bump. I slap on my widest fake smile, manage to yank off my cleated spinning shoe, and say, "Woot!" as a way of signaling *conversation over* but even as I do I have a sinking feeling that I'm about to be having more conversations like this everywhere—or at least more than usual. It's Paralympics time again.

Whenever the Games commence, the bodies of disabled athletes beam into living rooms everywhere, and for those nearly two weeks we are not described as "the disabled." No, we are overcomers. We are inspirations. We are superstars. We are heroes! We may even have theme songs.

I am not a Paralympian. Like all the other cyclists, I'm here because I have fitness goals. I buy magazines that promise "Your Best Body Yet!" I cycle because I'm vain. I like my miniskirts. But more than that, as a person with a disability, I'm playing the long game. This body is the only one I've got, and I need to take care of it.

Although Paralympians are getting the attention they have long deserved—more media coverage; more professional sponsorship and endorsements—the tenor of the conversation about these athletes and about disabled bodies in general makes it clear that they are misunderstood by most of the world and, save for this brief period, largely unseen.

During the Paralympic Games, it seems that we have sprung directly from the technological imagination of the 21st century. Those iron feet! Those wheelchair athletes and their superbuff biceps! But after the medals are awarded we retreat underground again—into normalcy, I guess, which is in fact a kind of oblivion when you have a body that is either an object of pity or valorized as "super" in order to be acceptable. It seems that, temporarily, able-bodied people make a virtue of their sudden awareness of disabled athletes. Truth is, we've been here all along.

I have been and have considered myself an athlete since the day I learned to ski at age 6 at the Winter Park Adaptive Ski Program in Winter Park, Colo., up until now, when I'm in the process of shaving minutes off my mile time. I'm tall; I like basketball. If

I'd had two real legs I would have kept up with ballet. But more than anything else, I like to be challenged physically, and I especially love dark, sweaty rooms where people scream "Go team!" or "Mind over matter!"

This would have been true, I believe, had I not lost my leg and lived and moved in a prosthesis for 40 years. But it's true now, and physical activity is a big—if not defining—part of my everyday life. It helps me keep up with my toddler, it makes me feel sexy for my sexy husband. Being athletic makes me *happy*. I don't want or need a medal for that.

My story is not inspirational; difficult at times, deeply sad at times, because I'm a flawed human being living in a flawed world, one in which women are often judged by their appearance above all else. I have not overcome my disability, and I never will. I will live with it for the rest of my life, and some days are better than others. Mine is an ordinary story to which anyone in any body should be able to relate.

But, as is so often the case, a nonnormative body must be made to be extraordinary, or what the sociologist Rebecca Chopp called "super-cripples": people who reach a level of physical performance that makes them seem "normal," their bodies palatable, acceptably different. People with disabilities can't be *just people*—a boundary between "us" and "them" must be established, if only to avoid the difficult truth that disability in some form will almost certainly touch their lives in the future.

My own life is not very exciting. Certainly not terribly exceptional. Does this make me a failed disabled person? Sometimes that's how it feels. But I am satisfied with being—in the words of a British friend—"quite sporty," a description I love, with its implications of buoyancy, ease, joy, a balance of beauty and strength, and especially ability. These adjectives are rarely (if ever) used to describe people with disabilities. I'll take them.

So although I watch those disabled athletes earn their props on the big stage, I also admit to being weary of having to get up on my own daily stage and field some embarrassing, prurient and occasionally soul-crushing questions. I'm an ordinary athlete living an ordinary life. I just happen to be doing it in a body many people might misunderstand, a body that is a source of pride and of shame, and sometimes, like all of our bodies on a good day, extraordinary.

The Hawk Can Soar

RANDI DAVENPORT

I PUSH THE WALKER IN FRONT OF ME, ITS FRONT WHEELS LARGER THAN the wheels in back. My right leg drags a little. My right foot drops. When I don't have the rollator in front of me—when I try to walk unaided—I have to bring my right hand up to my waist to create my own version of balance. Elbow clamped to my side. Stiffness where most other people have swing.

I'm also weak. Spastic. I wear braces for balance and support. How many times has some biotechnician cradled my feet in his or her hands, stroking the wrapping in place from which a new brace will be cast? I cannot count but I recall each time as if it were the same as the time before, the same as the time yet to come.

My hands quake with tremors, as do my father's hands and as did his father's hands before him. But I'm the lucky one. I'm the one who gets the disease, a rare form of motor neuron disease, in its full expression. My father and grandfather didn't even know they had a disease—*transmitted in an autosomal dominant pattern*, the geneticist said. They stopped being able to walk in their 70s and 80s and decided that this was caused by other things, perhaps by the nature of being old men, or a failure of the will to move, or the inconstant beating of their own blood.

It begins for me in my 30s. When I'm out running, my right foot goes out from under me, then comes back into position. It's nothing, I think. But over time, it happens more and more frequently. And other things come too, in silent waves: I stiffen like a tree trunk. I cannot easily rise from a chair. I cannot climb a flight of stairs. I cannot live my life without being overcome with profound fatigue, an exhaustion so deep and immeasurable that I weep when I don't have the strength to make dinner.

I tell myself that I'm working too hard. Trying to do too much. That all single parents are beset by weariness without end. I stop running and walk instead. When I can no longer walk any distance, I go to the gym. When I can no longer tolerate the gym, I go to the pool. But each new environment is a landscape of loss. What I could do and no longer can. What I can't do an irrefutable presence, as if lack has a shape and a weight.

A colleague at work points out my constant limp. I shrug. By this time, I have seen neurologists at Duke and Johns Hopkins. They're baffled. Something is wrong—on exam, my big toes point up, my reflexes jump, my muscles catch, my index finger shivers in a sign of a spinal lesion—but they can't say what. Only when I finally see a neuromuscular disease specialist at the big teaching hospital in Chapel Hill, N.C., do I find the doctor who knows what's gone wrong. In time, he delivers the news that I cannot be cured. I can only grow worse, my disability increasing in insidious increments that he will track by seeing me every three months.

Time passes. We watch, this doctor and I, as my disease moves through me. It's languid, quiet, but it moves. I grow weaker. I atrophy in discrete regions—my right foot and then my left and then my right hand—but I don't waste. I grow fat from immobility and then I grow thin again. I want to live as who I was, not as what this disease makes of me. This idea is a chimera but it helps me to think that I am fighting. I am a fighter. I always have been, even when I cannot win. At other times in my life, I might have viewed this as a pathological neurosis akin to tilting at windmills. Now I think of it as a saving grace. These tales I tell myself. The way I plan to escape fate. All to keep myself going.

Eventually, however, I am disabled. Disabled. Like this word is the sum total of my existence. That dragging leg. That dropping foot. That unbearable fatigue. A woman with a rollator moving

slowly through the world. These things signal my difference whenever I move. They are obvious. Unrestrained.

Soon, I leave my university career. I slowly begin to disappear
from view. The things I have earned seem ever further away. This
is the nature of this difference, I realize. The way disability stands
in for everything you were or ever would have been. Even when
you say it will not. Even when you refuse its existence. Disability is
contemptuous of your refusal. It scoffs at your desperate concern. It
pushes forward and it drags you after it.

I develop a serious side effect. A comorbidity, my doctors call it. I
nearly die. It doesn't matter that I said I would fight to stay upright.
It doesn't matter that I have resisted the wheelchair. My body has
other plans and it doesn't consult me. It is my own and yet it is
blind to my dreams. My desires. Weirdly, I begin to understand
that I am but a part of my body. My body is not a part of me.

Thus subordinated, I live. And I keep on living.

This story should end with an epiphany, a moment when I discover that I can still soar. How we love this narrative in America!
The ultimate act of bootstrapping: refusing to give in to a body you
cannot control and that medicine is helpless to cure.

And I nearly have such a moment. Leaning against my car in
a gas station by the side of a highway, pumping gas, I see a man
standing next to a pickup truck, an unremarkable sight save that
he has a huge hawk on his arm. The hawk is unblinded, its hood
draped over its neck like a collar, but it is lashed to the glove on the
man's arm like a dog to a post. Unaccountably, it sees me and tilts
its head and then tilts its head again.

What are you looking at? I think. As I so often think. But I wave
to the man and call, "Beautiful bird."

He nods and says they've been out hunting.

It's a dreary morning, mist hanging in veils over the fields, a
purplish tinge to the distant trees. I cannot imagine hunting in the
rain with a bird aloft but then I do. The rivulets of water standing in the farm ditches. The fresh scent of the pines. The breeze

lifting the sky and then lifting the sky again, each cloud turning. For just a moment, my heart lifts and, as if to answer me, the hawk rises and spreads its wings and then flaps back into place. Gives itself a shake as it strains against its bindings and then looks at me again, the expressionless light of its eyes seeming to say, What're you going to do?

Nothing, I say. I can do nothing.

I finish pumping my gas, and holding onto the side of my car for balance, I return the nozzle to its cradle, turn and climb back into the driver's seat and point my car south, toward home. A few minutes later, the man and the hawk are gone and nothing is left but the road ahead, occult, unknown, and yet so familiar by now that I feel every turn in my failing neurons. In my ever hopeful bones.

VI

LOVE

A Girlfriend of My Own

DANIEL SIMPSON

I PUT THE BITE OF WARM BALONEY SANDWICH BACK INTO THE LUNCH BAG with the half-eaten apple, then put the bag back into the southeast corner of my briefcase, the one I needed for carrying my bulky Braille books to and from school. My stomach felt unsettled. A cool, high tone—the progressive substitute for a bell—had sounded. I needed to get to Room 3 before it sounded again.

It was the spring of 1967. I had recently transferred to this suburban Philadelphia public high school with my identical twin brother, Dave, after 10 years at the Overbrook School for the Blind. We tried to fit in wherever we could. We went out for wrestling, played four-hand piano and sang in talent shows. We even threw a birthday party for ourselves, inviting some of the most popular and likable people in our class. There were awkward moments, but we did OK.

I had learned to walk with a white cane at Overbrook, but now that I had made the transition to public school, I refused to use it. Wasn't the rule to stay to the right, anyway? I shouldn't collide with anyone if we all followed the rules.

All the classrooms had their desks lined up in four rows of seven or eight. My desk in World Cultures was the second one down, second row from the door and the side chalkboard. I could navigate this way. I still remembered the location of my bed in the open dorm at the school for the blind, when I was 4—second one down in the row nearest the lockers.

Linda Fulton sat in the fourth seat from the front in the next row to the left. She spoke quietly, in a voice as smooth as the surfaces of our desks. In class—and in her presence—I tried to feel confident. I spoke up. I projected cool, even though I bet everyone could see through me.

A few years earlier, Jan and Dean recorded a song called "Linda." The minute I heard it, I knew I had to have it. But now that I knew *this* Linda, it had an even greater hold on me. Afternoons, when I got home from school, I played it again and again, singing along, extrapolating the slightest brush or interaction with her into something more.

I had something to say to Linda, to whom I spoke only occasionally, and then of things that had little importance. I wanted a girlfriend. I wanted one when I listened to the songs on WFIL while I got ready in the mornings and when we rode in the car and when my sister played the radio as she did the dishes and while I got ready for bed.

Once, when they let the boys and girls have gym class together during the unit on dance, I held Linda's hand and laughed with her as we tried to polka. She smelled of shampoo with a tinge of sweat. Her hand felt wider than I had imagined, wide and soft and relaxed. Being blind in this public school made my heart go a notch faster. *I could use a little softness*, I thought. *Relaxed would be good.*

I shimmied from my row to Linda's, trying to detect any book bags before I stepped right on them or made a fool of myself, tripping. I tried touching the edges of desks with the back of my hand as I shuffled backward, trying to look as normal as possible, not like a blind kid who needed to touch things.

"Hey, Dan, where are you going?"

"Right here," I said. "I was hoping to talk to you for a minute."

"Oh, yeah?"

"Ah—" My blood swished through my ears.

"Mr. Simpson, sit down, please. We're going to start." Mr. Coecher unpacked his briefcase and rustled some papers.

"In a few minutes," he said, "we're going to the auditorium for the presentation of awards, so we'll just spend 15 minutes or so on India."

"Can I walk up to the awards with you?" I whispered, angling back toward my desk. She didn't answer, but when I took my time packing up before we lined up to go, she stationed herself next to me and offered her hand.

Some people guide more naturally than others. They instinctively slow down at the beginning of a flight of stairs. They don't throw their arms out in front of your chest like some truck just cut them off and they're afraid you'll go flying through the windshield. I liked the ease with which she leaned into a right turn, away from my body, the way she gently crowded me to the left. I liked that the stairs were narrow enough that we had to press side against side to make room for traffic coming the other way. I didn't like how little time I had to ask my question:

"Linda, I like you. I just like you. I mean, you seem nice." This wasn't going the way I meant it to go.

"I was wondering if you'd go out with me, sometime."

After the sentence ran its way out of my mouth, it was like a fleet of skywriting planes had passed and I could hear the sound of surf again—the surf of everyone else talking and walking.

Linda let the surf roar for what seemed a long time. "I like you, too," she said, "but not in that way. You seem like a great guy but . . ."

For the awards ceremony, Linda sat to my right. Once we got to our seats, I had no reason, no excuse, to keep holding her hand. For a little while, she let our arms touch. Then, she moved hers from the armrest to her lap. I won a couple of awards, but they didn't mean that much. Something more important had just happened. I had walked with a sighted girl and asked for a date. She had turned me down with gentleness and honesty—maybe just like she would have turned down any other guy.

Love, Eventually

ONA GRITZ

ONE NIGHT WHEN I WAS VERY YOUNG, I LAY IN MY BED ACROSS FROM MY older sister's and described what I planned to look like when I grew up. My wavy brown hair would be straight and blond. My eyes, now the color of oversteeped tea, would turn blue. I wore a leg brace to bed in those days, a metal rod that buckled with a leather strap below my knee and attached to an ankle-high shoe. Though I felt the weight of this contraption as I spoke, and I knew I limped because the meanest girl on our block had told me, it went without saying that the beautiful future me would walk, and even run, with grace.

My sister listened without comment. She'd taught me to put pajama bottoms on my head so that when we danced like go-go girls it felt like we had long, swingy hair, and to dress our Barbies, with their shapely symmetrical legs, in fashionable outfits for their dates with G.I. Joe and Ken. The truest world I knew was the one she and I dreamed up. It made perfect sense to me that who we'd get to be in the mystical world of adulthood was completely up to us.

I have a form of cerebral palsy known as right hemiplegia, which essentially means only half my body is affected by the disability. My right limbs are tight, the muscles underdeveloped, and the fingers of that hand lack the dexterity and fine motor skills of those on my left. Years ago, I read an article about a rather new-age method for working with hemiplegic children. It suggested that while left hemiplegics respond well to straightforward instruction ("Raise your arm as best you can"), right hemiplegics do better with more poetic descriptions ("Imagine you're reaching for the stars"). This is due to differences between the left brain and right brain. Left hemiplegics have undamaged left hemispheres and tend to be pragmatic. But those of us with the right-side version depend on our undamaged, dreamy and artistic right hemispheres.

My cerebral palsy is relatively mild. I have clear speech, and though I walk slowly and awkwardly, I get around fine. In my 20s, if I considered my C.P. at all, it was through the lens of vanity. How noticeable was my limp? Was I pretty despite it? The answer, I assumed, was in the response I got from men. It was hard to decode. Apparently I was appealing enough to sleep with but not to be picked as a girlfriend.

Then I met a young man. He was handsome, athletic and crazy about me. We moved in together, got engaged, and my old habit of magical thinking surfaced. I believed his love canceled out my disability. Unfortunately, we had little in common. He liked the thrum and excitement of clubs. I preferred small gatherings and intimate conversation. He was happiest on a mountain bike. I was happiest at home with a book. Because of our disparate interests, we maintained largely separate social lives. I didn't actually mind this. My free time was given over to girlfriends, just like when I was single. Only now I had the perk of coming home to a handsome, affectionate man.

One of my closest friends was, and remains, a woman I came to know shortly before I was married. Hope was my first friend with cerebral palsy. Our connection was immediate and intense, fueled as it was by a sense of recognition that my imminent marriage lacked. I had other friends who "got me" in a visceral, finish-each-other's-sentences kind of way. But only Hope could finish the sentences I'd never before said aloud, the ones about how it felt to live in a non-normative body. Before we met, neither of us knew we craved those conversations, but we were starved for them. Though we share many interests, it would be weeks before we could tear ourselves away from the topic of disability long enough to discover what they were.

Without realizing it, I began to live a kind of split existence. By loving Hope I was learning to love a part of myself I'd deliberately ignored. Still, I continued to rely on the myth that being married to an able-bodied man meant I wasn't truly disabled. Only now do I see that he gave me a safe perch from which to peek at my identity as a disabled woman. I could take it on briefly, explore how it felt to claim it, and then go home to my real life. That is, my life of pretend.

Reality finally hit when we had a child. My husband eventually developed a very loving relationship with our son, but he wasn't exactly hands-on in the beginning. Before Ethan's birth I hadn't understood that parenting is physically demanding work. Caring for a newborn, especially, requires strength, balance and an ambidexterity I simply don't have. I couldn't bathe Ethan safely, carry him on stairs or even sip from a water glass while he nursed if his head rested on my good arm. Finally, I was forced to acknowledge that my C.P. is more than a cosmetic issue. Some tasks I could manage by making adaptations, but for many I needed to ask for help.

At first, I felt deeply embarrassed by what I perceived as my ineptitude. But at some point, while I was busy figuring out ways to get the work done, I forgot about the shame.

By the time Ethan turned 3, the physical demands of mothering had lessened and I could focus on the parts that came easily— talking with him, reading together, entering into his imaginary worlds. A year later, my husband and I divorced. Thankfully, by then I understood that my tie to him wasn't what made me whole.

In a long-ago interview with Bill Moyers, Maya Angelou revealed her theory that most women marry other people's husbands. She didn't elaborate, but I immediately understood. Out of hopefulness, impatience, insecurity or for a thousand other reasons, we too often rush into relationships that are poor fits for us, robbing our partners and ourselves of more promising connections. It struck me as likely that those of us with disabilities are especially susceptible to this.

"I have finally married my own husband," Ms. Angelou went on to say. Many years after my first marriage, so did I. Dan and I met in a poetry workshop.

"Of course," Hope said, when I told her that my new love was not only a fellow writer, but someone with a disability. "It's like you guys are the same person, only one's male and one's female," said Ethan—not entirely as a compliment—who was 8 at the time.

It's true that Dan and I are very similar. We're both romantics yet also fiercely independent. We're introspective to the point of obsession. Though he's a decade older, we share a love for the music from his teenage years. And long before we met, many of the same novels and poetry books lined our shelves.

As for our disabilities, they're nothing alike. Dan was born blind, and that library of his is largely in Braille and audio. He sees light, but no shapes or objects.

"Does the light have a color?" I asked when first getting to know him. But, of course, since light is all he can see, he has no way to know.

Dan confided to me that back in high school and college, he knew how to use a cane but chose to walk without one in an attempt to blend in. Back then, he also sought able, sighted women rumored to be beautiful. When I shared my stories in kind, I was struck, just as I'd once been with Hope, by how little had to be explained. Clearly, though our disabilities are different, the emotions and their residue are much the same.

These days, disability is a mere factor in our daily routines. It's there when I need to proofread Dan's Word documents for formatting inconsistencies or tell him which bottle contains Tylenol and which the dog's allergy meds, just as it is when he has to climb ladders to change our smoke alarm batteries or hold me upright as we walk on ice-slick streets. I read the mail to Dan, of course, but also poems and stories. He reads to me too, running his fingers along pages of Braille as though skimming them through water. And yes, his touch on my skin is just as attentive and skilled.

Disability has also earned a central place in our creative work. We've both written extensively about living in these particular bodies of ours, and spoken at universities and on panels about disability poetics. Many of our friends are artists and writers with disabilities. It's a rich life, one I never could've imagined despite my famously active imagination.

Still, had the possibility of this loving bi-disability marriage presented itself to us years earlier, I don't think either of us would have been ready. We needed the right combination of fallacies, wrong turns and formative relationships to lead each of us exactly here.

How to Play the Online Dating Game, in a Wheelchair

EMILY LADAU

THE FIRST TIME I FORAYED INTO ONLINE DATING, I LET MY WHEEL-chair show just a little in my photos. The good guys, I hoped, would be so taken by my clever profile and witty banter that they'd be able to look beyond my disability, if they even noticed it at all.

I eagerly began swiping, quickly matching with an attractive man whose profile picture showed him sporting an enormous iguana on his shoulder. Thinking that would make for an easy conversation starter, I messaged him. A few minutes later, he replied, but instead of responding to my reptilian inquiry, he asked, "Are you in a wheelchair?"

I kept my answer simple and told him that yes, I do use a wheelchair, but I was much more interested in the back story of the iguana. Unfortunately, he wasn't interested at all, messaging back only to say: "Sorry. The wheelchair's a deal-breaker for me."

His blunt reply stung, but the feeling was nothing new. Because I was born with my disability—Larsen syndrome, a genetic joint and muscle disorder—I'd already gathered a pile of romantic rejections seemingly big enough to fill an Olympic swimming pool by the time I downloaded Tinder. This particular rejection, however, unleashed a wave of panic within me.

A few months before my initial swipes, I'd gone through a messy breakup with a man I dated for over two years. I truly believed he was the person I'd marry, and that I'd never have to worry about rejection again. When I found myself newly single, I turned to online dating in the hopes of easing my fears that no one else would ever accept me as I am, that lightning doesn't strike twice.

Not one to be deterred, I persevered, downloading every possible dating app and creating accounts on various dating sites. But I became skittish about revealing my disability, because in an already shallow dating culture, I believed my wheelchair would cause most men to write me off without a second thought. So I decided to hide my disability completely. I cropped my wheelchair out of my photos. I eliminated any mention of it in my profiles. In this virtual world, I could pretend my disability didn't exist.

I kept up with this facade for a while, messaging matches who were none the wiser. Once I thought I'd spoken with a guy long enough to establish his interest, I'd choose a moment to strike, telling him about my disability. I'd send a long-winded explanation divulging my wheelchair use, reminding him that it didn't make me any less of a person and ending with reassurance that he could ask me questions, should he have any.

After dropping the "wheelchair bomb," I'd have to brace myself for their reactions, which were always a mixed bag, often ranging from indifference to ghosting. Occasionally, I'd receive an accepting response.

One man that I connected with on Coffee Meets Bagel was incredibly apologetic when I first told him about my wheelchair, as though it was the most tragic thing he'd ever heard. I shut that down by explaining that my disability is part of who I am and it's nothing to be sorry for. I ended up going on one date with him, and then another. For the second date, my bagel suggested a painting night (a social event that involves paintbrushes, canvases, acrylics and, usually, wine) since I'd told him how much I enjoy them. He found a Groupon and I researched a location, picking out a restaurant in New York City that was supposed to be wheelchair accessible.

As it turned out, the restaurant was accessible, but the painting class was happening in a room upstairs. So, we spent our entire date sitting directly below the painters, eating dinner and making strained conversation with wine-fueled laughter and painting instruction in the background. I was mortified. Following that disaster, I promised my date I'd get his money back. As soon as the company refunded our tickets, I never heard from him again.

It was painful to realize that the hard part isn't over once someone learns that I'm disabled. Going on dates with me can be a crash course on disability, and I recognize that's not always easy for non-disabled people to process. But I wasn't helping the situation by keeping the existence of my disability concealed, springing it upon people only when I thought it felt right. In retrospect, this served only to contribute to the stigma I usually work so hard to fight.

I felt like a hypocrite. In every other area of my life, my disability is front and center. I write and speak endlessly about being a proud, unapologetic disabled woman. It is part of my identity, shaping everything I do and everything I value. But in the online dating world, my disability was my secret shame.

So I decided it was time for a change. I started gradually, making references to my disability throughout my profile, then adding photos in which my wheelchair is clearly visible. I tried to keep things light and humorous. For instance, OKCupid asks users to list six things they can't live without; one of mine is "the invention of the wheel."

Still, I found myself having to make sure that potential matches had actually picked up on the trail of clues I'd left. I grew tired of feeling like I needed to deceive men into being interested because society instilled in me that my disability makes me undesirable. Finally, I took the leap I'd been so afraid to make, opening up about disability to strangers whom I hoped would appreciate my honesty and perhaps send me a message.

Prominently in my profile, I wrote: "I'd like to be very upfront about the fact that I use a wheelchair. My disability is part of my identity and I'm a loud, proud disability rights activist, but there is so much more that defines me (you know, like the stuff I've got in my profile). I realize some people are hesitant to date a human who experiences the world sitting down. But I'd like to think you'll keep reading and dive a little deeper. And you're welcome to ask questions, should you have any."

Once I added that paragraph, I felt liberated, relieved that anyone I spoke to would have a clearer picture of me. There have been plenty of matches that haven't worked out, and whether that's actually because of my disability, I'll never know. But I had a nearly yearlong relationship with a man I met through OKCupid, so I know it's possible for lightning to strike again. My dating life remains a comedy of errors, and I still struggle every day with the feeling that my disability means I won't find love, but at least I'm being true to myself. I'm putting myself out there—my whole self—and it feels good to be proud of who I am.

Explaining Our Bodies, Finding Ourselves

MOLLY McCULLY BROWN AND SUSANNAH NEVISON

IN JULY OF 2016 MOLLY MCCULLY BROWN AND SUSANNAH NEVISON MET for the first time at the Sewanee Writers' Conference in Tennessee. As working poets with physical disabilities, a condition each explores in her work, they found much in common and quickly became friends, and have grown closer over time. These essays make up a dialogue about being disabled in an able-bodied world that arose from their friendship.

Calling Long Distance

There's SO MUCH standing at this party. Legs are the worst, I hate them!

I send this text from a corner of my university's beginning-of-the-year department get-together, leaning heavily on my cane and trying to arrange my face in such a way that I don't look too uncomfortable. Our department chair's house is up two shallow flights of brick stairs, and anyway, even if I could get my wheelchair inside, the whole place is packed to the gills with people and I could never move in it.

Instead, I make do relying on walls and various pieces of furniture for support. Periodically, I perch for a few minutes on the couch, but no one stays sitting long, and from down there, it's impossible to hear anyone who's standing over the din. The expectation is that you'll circulate.

I love my colleagues, and I'm happy to see them, but every year I *hate* this party. There comes a point a little way into the evening when the pain in my knees and back and ankles reaches a roaring point and my head is filled with the sound of a false ocean, as if my ear is pressed to the mouth of a conch shell.

I can only half-concentrate on what anyone is saying to me. They're all muted, and my brain is busy balancing and breathing. The truth about pain is that it makes you tired. My body needs to rest, but it's more than that. I'm exhausted by having to feign comfort, and I don't want to translate what's going on inside me, even for my friends. They're sorry when I'm hurting, but for them, the act of rising from the couch and standing is effortless and instant. All that explaining my body will do is widen the gulf between us.

Usually, this is the point where I take myself off to the side for a moment and sit down apart from everyone. This year, though, my phone chimes quietly and brightly in my hand—

I was just thinking the same thing! THE WORST! Lots of standing here, too.

Susannah, a friend and fellow poet, who also has a physical disability, is texting from her own department party across the country, in Utah. Susannah and I publish with the same press, but we hadn't met until this summer, when by chance we ended up at the same writer's conference. She found me the first night, and we fell in like we'd known each other forever, trading medical histories so extensive that one woman, shocked to overhear us, yelped, "You two are falling apart!" We laughed until we couldn't breathe. And since we've gone home to our separate states, we've spoken almost every day.

You're falling apart. This is a version of a truth I've known about myself ever since I can remember: *Your name is Molly. You have curly hair. You like to talk. You're falling apart.* The medical version of the matter goes like this: As a result of being born prematurely and deprived of oxygen, I have cerebral palsy, a neurological disorder. My particular type increases my muscle tone and hinders my balance. I can walk, but only a little. I can stand, but not for long. My crouched, spastic gate puts too much pressure on my joints and so the cartilage in my knees and ankles is wearing away. I am, quite literally, falling apart, even if it is at a relatively glacial pace.

This fact was delivered, first, in the mouths of doctors talking over my head to my parents about possible surgical and orthopedic interventions: selective dorsal rhizotomy, partial hamstring release, heel cord lengthening, double-upright-KFOs. Then I heard it in the mouths of the people who loved me, trying to give me the tools to live the rest of my life as painlessly and independently as possible: *I know it hurts, but you have to stretch, you have to walk, you have to put weight on your legs. Otherwise, you won't be able to walk anymore.* If you aren't walking, I learned from the world, your body's no good.

Somewhere along the way, I got cleaved down the middle. There was my damaged body, and then there was the rest of me, desperately trying to hold that body together, thinking: *I hate you* and then *I need you* and then *thank you* and then *please don't fall apart!*

These days, a lot of the language I use about my own life still reflects that split. I'm visibly disabled, and so I have to talk about my body everywhere I go. Sometimes, it's to assuage people's curiosity: The woman in the shoe store wants to know what happened to me, or the man I'm on a first date with hasn't asked about my family but is weirdly hungry for details about just what *exactly* my body can do, just how *exactly* I'm scarred. Sometimes, explaining is a matter of necessity: I need to know if there's an elevator in the building where I teach this semester.

Sometimes, I'm not sure exactly why it is I'm explaining: On the first day of the new semester I ask my students if they have any questions about me, and one boy puts up a hand and asks, utterly guileless: *So, what is it that's wrong with you?* I'm a relatively new teacher, and this hasn't happened to me before. Still, I answer him the way I've grown accustomed to answering. *I have a disability,* I say, like it's a shirt I put on in the morning. *It makes my balance bad. It means I don't walk very well.* After that, we have a conversation about why, in a writing class especially, being careful and exacting with our language is so important, but I can't stop that exchange from pinging around in my skull.

The truth is that even with the people who know and love me best, I have a nasty habit of treating my body like it's a bad suit of clothes or a thing that somehow just keeps *happening* to me. I don't talk much about it unless I need to explain: *I can't do this* or *Could you give me a hand with that* or *I'm sorry, I can't go there.* Mostly, I try to render it background noise. *Sometimes I forget you have a disability,* a friend says. An ex-boyfriend said once: *It's such a small thing.* I did this on purpose. Their forgetting is my most impressive magic trick.

I never forget about my disability—its root system is shot through every part of me. This is true on a basic biological level: It's a feature of my brain and the electrical signals it sends. But I mean it more deeply than that. It's not just that I'm often in pain, or that I have to think about my body almost all the time, although both of these things are true. It's that *I don't exist* without my body. Its particular margins, and movements and methods for making it through the world are present, not just in the moments when it causes me hardship but in the best and wildest and strongest stretches of my being. My body isn't standing apart from me holding my life in a vise grip: It is *making* my life, indivisible from the rest of me. We are walking together through the world, as odd and slow as it looks.

I hate my legs, and I don't. I love my body, and I don't. There is a list of things that are wrong with me, and none of them are wrong with me. I go whole stretches of time without pausing to think: *I have a disability.* I am always, always, always disabled. When I make my life legible to an able-bodied world, all the nuance, all those contradictions, which aren't really contradictions, get sucked out of it, somehow. Even I start to forget them. Any way you slice it, explaining is an act of erasure. Either I am describing my body so that it can be understood and thereby forgotten: *Look, it's not so scary after all—there it goes settling down in the corner to sleep.* Or I am describing my body so that it begins to subsume the rest of me: *Look, she grows curiouser and curiouser—that wheelchair, that weird walk, that way her hands curl up.*

Susannah and I are on the phone in the middle of a slow Tuesday and I can't stop thinking how weirdly grateful I feel for her voice on the other end of the line. We're talking about our bodies, and then not about our bodies, about her dog, and my classes, and the zip line we'd like to string between us, from Mississippi all the way to Utah. And then we're talking about our bodies again, that sense of being both separate and not separate from the skin we're in. And it hits me all at once that none of this is in translation, none of this is *explaining. Legs are the worst,* I say, *I hate them.* And I know she knows I mean it, but that I also mean: *I love them* and *I'm grateful* and *I'm glad you're here.* I also mean *I'm tired.* And I also mean *thank God.*

—Molly McCully Brown

Lost (and Found) in Translation

A few years ago, I started going to a new indoor pool. As soon as I had stripped down to my bathing suit in the dressing room, a woman asked, "What happened to you? Were you in some kind of accident?" Like the student in Molly's class, this woman asked me to explain my body. I wanted to simply say no, I was not in an accident, but I've spent a good part of my life making people more comfortable with my body, and offered my prepared translation. Without even thinking, I said, "I've had a lot of surgery."

To be asked to account for my body, especially by strangers, reminds me that my body needs its own introduction, that it visually disrupts or upsets another person's field of vision. My body requires explanation in public spaces because public spaces aren't made for people who look like me.

As long as I can remember, I've been taught to speak about disability as something that exists in addition to myself. I'd say *I was born with extensive birth defects in my legs and feet.* I'd say *I have a lot of foot and leg issues.* At no point would I have said *I'm disabled.* Undoubtedly, this semantic dislocation is related to the fact that I can render disability invisible. If I wear pants, no one sees the scars. To the untrained eye, I walk normally. I have the privilege of passing as completely able-bodied in appearance, if not in practice. This point might seem small, but it isn't. Growing up, I thought I could be in possession of physical disabilities without being physically disabled. Because I could pass for able-bodied, I could perform some kind of normalcy. I could put disability away like a costume; I could take it on and off.

Explaining disability is like speaking two languages, and it is the disabled person who is required to translate for the able-bodied world. Can I refuse to translate? It doesn't feel like an option. A refusal to translate is a refusal to turn the elephant in the room into a mouse. But this is what the world around me asks me to do, and more often than not I oblige. Still, this mouse has the power to terrorize me.

I learned very early on to advocate for myself, to take ownership of my body. I'd rattle off the terms: *bilateral club foot. A leg-length discrepancy. Congenital birth defects.* Precision in language grants narrative power. So long as I could name it, I could explain it, and in a way control it. I could reframe the way I was seen.

And yet, so often the act of naming disability enables another person to look away, or refuse to see me as I am. I move in an instant from a hypervisible object of curiosity to an invisible nonentity.

I often think of my body, and disability, as an object I command, or try to command. Language shapes how I understand myself—I am both my disability and the mind that needs to exist apart from it. I am always dual. This division of self, or the need to perform that division in language, is something I unwittingly learned from the medical model, as I listened to doctors discuss *her deformity* or *her birth defects* with my parents. I also understand my body as a made object.

The body I was born with, as Molly pointed out on the phone the other day, *wasn't going to work out so well*. The body I live in is the product of many hands: I move through the world in a vessel that was given to me, that was shaped and reshaped through surgery, so that I can propel myself through space and time without the need for a wheelchair. It is both mine and not mine. I have never consciously known my body as it entered the world. It's a strange kind of grief I carry, a weird nostalgia not for something better, but for some truer version of myself. As if to know my original body would somehow move me closer to an understanding of that split I—as if maybe then I would be one and not two, disability a nameable part of me instead of something I hold beside me.

Moments like the one in the pool dressing room, moments where I can see the instant someone registers my body as deviant, force that complicated relationship with disability to the foreground. The removal of sweatpants in a dressing room is the removal of an able-bodied facade. It forces the linguistic toggle between *I'm disabled* and *I have a disability.*

When my body misbehaves, as it inevitably does, that distinction between being disabled and having a disability becomes shaky, and shakier still when repeated surgical intervention is warranted. Then, disability is no longer something I command, hide or control. It eclipses me. It becomes a defining characteristic. Under a stranger's gaze, I become the woman on crutches or the woman in the wheelchair. In other people's eyes, I'm clearly disabled. Whether I like it or not, it's impossible to completely separate body and self. In terms of pronouns, *we* have to figure out how to be *me*. We have to work as one.

Unlike when I remove sweatpants in a dressing room, there's no point when disability isn't present for me. Though I perform that division in speech, in explaining disability, I'm always aware of myself as disabled. I'm always thinking, consciously, about how I move. If I don't, I stumble. For any major life event, I can tell you what shoes I was wearing and what kinds of surfaces I walked on, whether the cement was cracked, how big the gravel was. I plan my day around how much walking I'll do, and whether it will be flat or on an incline. Why then is it so hard for me to say *I'm disabled?*

Perhaps part of it comes from the near-constant performance of able-bodiedness. Perhaps part of it is that I've adapted so well, and I've made such progress in the eyes of the medical field. Perhaps I really do believe that I can separate my body from my self, because I do it all the time in language.

When I found out Molly was at the writers' conference, I made a beeline for her table and introduced myself. Within minutes, we were laughing and sharing hospital stories. There was no explaining, no need for back story. No need to define ourselves or our bodies. There was simply the joy of being recognized, that rare and easy space, where there is never any need for translation.

—Susannah Nevison

Longing for the Male Gaze

JENNIFER BARTLETT

WHEN I WAS IN MY EARLY 30s, I PRACTICED YOGA AT A STUDIO IN my neighborhood in Brooklyn. On most days, I walked there with two friends—one who was in her 20s and one about my age—but occasionally we each got to class on our own. There was a construction site across the street as part of the growing onslaught of gentrification in the neighborhood. My friends would often complain about being harassed and catcalled by the construction workers—even more so when they wore their yoga clothes. I passed the site day after day without incident.

When I was younger, in my 20s, I was a thin, slight woman. I have also always been beautiful and a nice dresser. I also happen to have cerebral palsy, which affects my motor skills, balance and speech, as it does with most people who have it. It is typically caused by damage to or malformation of the brain during birth or infancy. In my case, my mother's umbilical cord was wrapped around my neck in utero. As my mother was unable to have an emergency cesarean section, I was strangled by the cord, and born clinically dead. The temporary lack of oxygen caused damage to a portion of my brain.

Cerebral palsy is not uniform and manifests in a number of ways. It might affect all limbs severely, or just one side of the body; or the effects may be slight, making the disability barely perceptible. It can affect strength, balance and movement; some with the condition may not be able to walk unassisted or care for themselves in typical ways.

To put it bluntly, people with cerebral palsy appear to have strange movements. Since they are not in full control of their muscles, they may have facial expressions or spasticity that most people find surprising, if not unattractive.

People with cerebral palsy are often mistaken for having a mental impairment, although the two are not necessarily linked. I have a speech impediment and awkward gait. My disability is visible, but not necessarily significant. I do have some physical limitations, but am able to do most things that a typical person can do. My primary difficulty has been with people's negative reaction, or what disability-studies scholars call the "social construction" of disability. This primarily means that the main challenges disabled people face come from societal prejudice and inaccessible spaces.

Recently, the popular feminist Jessica Valenti published a memoir titled "Sex Object," which focuses on the toll the "male gaze" has taken on her. She wrote an article on this theme for this paper, "What Does a Lifetime of Leers Do to Us?" Ms. Valenti describes a life of sexual harassment beginning at adolescence. She writes of what seems like countless instances of men exposing themselves to her on the New York City subway. She describes constantly thwarting unwanted advances from men in all areas of her life. Ms. Valenti currently has a 5-year-old daughter, and she wrestles for a way to prepare her child for an onslaught of male harassment. She takes for granted that this will happen.

My experiences have been quite different, nearly the opposite, of Ms. Valenti's and that of most women. I was never hit on or sexually harassed by my professors in college, or later, by my coworkers or superiors. I have not felt as if my male teachers, friends or colleagues thought less of me because of my gender. I've never been aggressively "hit on" in a bar, despite the fact that I have frequented them alone throughout the years. In fact, I've rarely been approached in a bar at all.

I do remember being sexually harassed by a man on the street. Once. I was 18 years old. I was waiting for a bus, and a man pulled up and offered me a ride in his car. When I declined, he got hostile and asked me if I was wearing panties. I was more startled than anything, and I left the curb to go to the nearby movie theater where my friend worked. I didn't tell my friend what happened, but waited with him for the bus. This was very frightening, but I wouldn't say the incident traumatized me, nor is it something that deeply affected my life. And it happened only once.

Let me rephrase that: It happened only once while I was visibly inhabiting my own body. Virtually, it has been another story.

In 2013, I began experimenting with the dating website OKCupid because I wanted to explore this concept of being desexualized. I created a provocative profile. The photographs were recent, but in photographs, I look "normal." I did not mention that I have cerebral palsy. I wanted to use the opportunity to explore the sexual world as an able-bodied woman, if only online, and see what all the fuss was about.

As a pretend, able-bodied woman, I received all kinds of messages. Men wrote stupid things, aggressive things and provocative things. Often, while I was in a dialogue with a man who didn't know of my impairment, I would disclose it, and almost always, the man vanished, no matter how strong the connection had been beforehand.

After a while, I changed the profile to reflect that I have a disability. Fewer men wrote. Sometimes, no men wrote, depending on the content. But overall, the messages changed. They could be called more respectful. The men who wrote primarily wanted to know how my disability affected me.

This all feels like a political act, and in some ways it is. Strangely, my disability makes me feel as if I have license to play with and deconstruct sexuality in ways I might not have the bravery to do as an able-bodied woman.

I watch men on the street. I will watch a man visually or verbally harass women who pass him. I am invisible enough to do this. Sometimes men look at me, but the reaction is different. There seems to be some level of shame or confusion mixed with the lust in their eyes. Does this mean that I am lucky? Am I blessed to be sexually invisible and given a reprieve from something that has troubled women for centuries?

It certainly does not *feel* that way. On one hand, I know that I am "lucky" not to be sexually harassed as I navigate the New York City streets. But I am harassed in other ways that feel much more damaging. People stare. People insist that I have God's blessing. People feel most comfortable speaking about me in the third person rather than addressing me directly. It is not uncommon that I will be in a situation where a stranger will talk to the nearest able-bodied person, whether it be a friend or a complete stranger, *about me* to avoid speaking *to* me.

I also do understand what it feels like to get attention from the wrong man. It's gross. It's uncomfortable. It's scary and tedious. And in certain cases, traumatic. But I still would much rather have a man make an inappropriate sexual comment than be referred to in the third person or have someone express surprise over the fact that I have a career. The former, unfortunately, feels "normal." The latter makes me feel invisible and is meant for that purpose.

I *like* it when men look at me. It feels empowering. Frankly, it makes me feel like I'm not being excluded.

Intimacy Without Touch

ELIZABETH JAMESON AND CATHERINE MONAHON

ONE OF MY OLDEST FRIENDS IS HERE TO VISIT. FOR AS LONG AS WE'VE known each other, we've been in sync, weaving in and out of each other's lives and reaching milestones together. We married our partners around the same time, went through law school and medical school at the same time, got pregnant with our sons in unison and lived as neighbors for years. Although we have visited each other frequently, time has slowly gotten away from us. I haven't seen her in more than a year.

She gingerly lies down on the sofa while I sit nearby. She isn't looking good. Thinner than I've ever seen her, weak and in pain. "How are you?" I ask.

"Well, I have cancer," she says plainly. She changes the subject, not feeling the need to linger on her recent prognosis or to specify that it is terminal. All I want to do is hold her hand, rub her shoulders and tell her how much she means to me with a firm, loving touch. I stay distant from her, unable to move. I imagine stroking her hair or giving her a pillow to feel more comfortable, but I cannot do anything. Our conversation ebbs, flows, then trickles into silence; there is not much more to say.

She rests her hands on her stomach, where she holds the most pain. Five years ago, I would have bridged this silence with a gentle hug or touch. But I am stuck, immobile, unable to express my thoughts and feelings. I don't allow myself to cry as we say our goodbyes.

When I lost the use of my hands, I lost my love language. I have multiple sclerosis, which has resulted in the loss of the use of my limbs. My disease progresses so slowly that I am caught by surprise when I can no longer do something. Little did I know I have been losing my range of motion by a fraction of a centimeter every day. Nerve by nerve, I lost the use of my legs, arms, wrists, hands, pointer finger, thumb.

I can't tell you when exactly I became a quadriplegic, only that I know I am now a part of the club. My paralysis limits me down to my fingertips. I can't operate my wheelchair, can't hold a coffee cup, let alone someone's hand—I can't actively touch in any way. Like a fortress, my wheelchair is both impossible to leave and difficult to enter. If others want to reach out and touch me, it can be intimidating to make the first move. It feels like there is a thick pane of glass separating me from the outside world, and because of my physical disability, I begin to believe that I am powerless to break through.

Over the years, I have tried to make a home out of my fortress, my glass bubble, uncomfortably settling into my grief. There are times when I feel connected to others, but in most situations, I become passive. I work hard to forget the joy of touching. *I am a positive person*, I tell myself, *I can deal with this.* I set up camp at the base of my Mount Everest and try not to glance up at what I am missing.

But I feel the loss of touch as if it were a limb that has been severed from my body, an invisible, open wound I painstakingly cover up each day. I am hyperaware of the moments when words are not enough. When touching someone's hand is the only way I can truly communicate my feelings. When I can't greet someone familiar by warmly placing my hand on their shoulder. Or when I know someone is sad, and it's not appropriate to talk about what's wrong; I can't reassure them affectionately. It is like not being able to breathe. This loss, in combination with the guilt I feel when I grieve it, is overwhelming. I resign myself to the idea that I will never experience consensual, nourishing, intimate exchanges of touch in everyday life.

It is in this state of numbed resignation that an unexpected crack forms in the thick glass that has been separating me from "normal" people: A ray of light that reveals a world of intimacy I have been overlooking.

I am visiting with another friend at a coffee shop. My voice is weak and hard to hear in crowded spaces, so I use a voice amplifier. The amplifier has a microphone and a headset that make me look like an aerobics instructor who happens to be teaching in a wheelchair. I've got my headset in place, but when my friend leans in to hear me, it's no use. My voice is too faint. I motion with my head toward the dial on the device, which can be turned up to make my voice louder. He tentatively discovers the dial, locking eyes with me to check the loudness of my voice. As I keep talking, he turns the dial up, then up and up some more until, *yes, there*, he can hear me. We nod and smile in unison, return to our conversation.

As he settles back into his chair, I feel lightheaded. By increasing the volume of my voice, he had turned up the very essence of "me." The fact that he cared so much to hear me. That he took the time to learn how to connect with me.

I had rediscovered intimacy, without touch.

My mind continued to reel long after we said our goodbyes. *Maybe I can experience intimacy*, I thought. *It's just that the language of it all has just changed.* I had to redefine intimacy for myself. What is it, without touch? The freedom to express myself. The joy of being recognized, seen, accepted, equal. Letting my guard down, no longer burdened by society's version of me, by my version of me. The feeling when the stigmas of disability and illness are lifted. I eyed my version of Mount Everest, thinking that maybe there was a way for me to fully rejoin the living.

After that day in the coffee shop, intimate moments emerged from the fabric of my everyday life. I began to notice how friends, loved ones and total strangers could make me feel visible and whole in completely mundane ways. Appreciating them took my breath away: that someone driving my wheelchair is making love to me, that someone kneeling to my eye level is giving me a gentle caress, that someone feeding me is a joint experience of pleasure and tenderness.

Within the mundane there are beautiful surprises, too. On a busy day, before work, my husband pauses his morning routine to make me a poached egg, his specialty. Something he wants to make for me—I didn't ask. A friend tries to feed me a cookie. He does it "wrong" at first, but the process of figuring out the best way is like an intricate dance. Over the holidays, a family member puts on Handel's "Messiah," music that I love and everyone else in the family finds annoying. They usually refuse to put it on, but this morning they play it just for me, blasting it so that I can hear the music through my bedroom wall.

I savored these moments, and as I did I was propelled and empowered by them. I realized I could play an active role—I could give as well as receive. So I took my intimacy into my own hands, even though I am still grieving what I cannot do. I leave base camp behind and begin my slow, labored ascent; the fluid, open concept of intimacy spurs me onward.

I have always loved food. I muster the courage to ask someone to join me for a luxurious, two-hour pastry-eating session. We take the time to savor every crumb of a single pastry, eating at the same pace together, and I feel honored, loved.

I start seeing myself in others: I am a part of a tribe. Wheelchair users, people with multiple sclerosis, the elderly with canes and walkers, people struggling with aphasia or spinal cord injury. The list goes on and on. We are everywhere. I lock eyes with a 90-year-old man in a crowded elevator. He tips his hat to me with a warm smile. I see a woman with a mobility aide in the street and we grin at each other, comrades. Neighbors. Strangers. Visible, invisible.

I poke fun at my own disability, creating humor where there was once shame. When I'm drinking water, I have no way to stop, so when someone cracks a joke I laugh and spit water down my front. It's humiliating, but hysterically funny at the same time. I have a damp front more often than not.

I now know intimacy can be everywhere. Moments I've noticed, received, created. You and I are sharing an intimate moment right now—because if you've gotten this far without turning away, you are a part of that exclusive tribe of people who truly see me.

But eventually, my quest for intimacy brings me back to the beginning. To touch.

My good friend is back to visit. We are trying to see each other more often—with less time left, it's only natural. She lies on the sofa, and I verbalize all that I kept inside last time—how badly I want to stroke her hair, squeeze her hand, sit next to her. She smiles appreciatively, but moves the conversation along, not one to linger in the spotlight. She directs the conversation back to me.

We talk a bit more, and emboldened by my confession, I ask her if she would take my hand, if it isn't too painful to move. Slowly, she sits up, and my caregiver rolls my chair as close to her as possible. She extends her hand, resting it in mine. We look at each other and breathe.

The Three-Legged Dog
Who Carried Me

LAURIE CLEMENTS LAMBETH

THE VETERINARIAN KNELT OVER MY THREE-LEGGED AUSTRALIAN shepherd, Patou, in my living room. She had just completed the procedure to end Patou's life. The first injection was to relax her; my husband and I, holding her, felt her taut back muscles melt into a softness we hadn't known for years. The second vial sent her off.

"Now she'll be whole again, reunited with her other leg," the doctor said.

I knew what she meant about *wholeness*: It was a belief in an embodied afterlife. Born with four legs yet living the last years of her life with three, Patou must have seemed to some incomplete. But in that moment I had to question that idea.

In the four and a half years after Patou's initial bone cancer diagnosis (fibrosarcoma) and the amputation of her front leg, she became more herself than ever before—committed to the joy of any small moment, growing less introverted and more trusting with outsiders, and, like most dogs lucky enough to live into their golden years, developing ever deeper bonds with the people who cared for her.

Even more, through our shared experience of disability—she with three legs, I often with my "third leg," a cane—we grew all the more connected through our interdependence, our unconventional mobility and our asymmetry.

When Patou came into my life, I had lived with relapsing-remitting multiple sclerosis for almost nine years, which caused periods of numbness, dizzy spells and weakness on my left side that impaired my mobility. I had collected three canes by then. Aware that a flare-up could come at any time without notice, I taught the young, four-legged Patou to help me up stairs.

Aussies are herding dogs and need a job of some kind, and she loved hoisting me up stairs—actually, any nearby stairway—heaving her whole body for us both through short, rolling bounds. With one hand I would hold the rail and with the other I grasped her collar, and she pulled me up, surging. Like a cane, she took the strain off, but steadied as I went. It strikes me only now, as I write this, how similar that motion on four legs was to her movement years later on three: the absolute effort and drive of that round-backed, full body propulsion.

Couldn't that be wholeness? Might we store all our past and future ways of moving within us at all times?

I also trained Patou to pull me up in case I fell, and to stand still beside me as I attempted to rise from a seated position, holding her sturdy back for stability.

My potential need became her game.

Many MS flares have come and gone since then, leaving their residual effects along the way. A few months before Patou displayed symptoms of bone cancer, my right eye flamed a deep pain with movement and the glare of bright light, and I soon lost the ability to read most text for about a year, the letters rising up out of themselves: MS-related optic neuritis. Just as I contemplated a different life of listening more than reading, of possibly needing a larger dog to help me navigate the world, Patou began needing me more.

At an agility class the summer before the cancer diagnosis, she ran up a tall wooden apex structure called an A-frame, and couldn't make it to the top. She stopped a little higher than my shoulders, unable to gather enough momentum to climb all the way up the steep incline, and she turned to me. This was the moment my dog let me know that she needed me. I stretched out my arms, watching

her scramble to gain footing, and she dropped into them, unchar-
acteristically laying each front paw on either side of my neck.

It felt like wholeness, holding this 45-pound dog like a child, but
tentative. What is wholeness?

All bodies change over time; no one body is ever permanent
or completely symmetrical. After her amputation, Patou's body
remolded itself to suit her movement. Her solitary front paw, the
left one, angled inward, forming a strong center paw. It grew to
nearly twice its original size, eventually capable of holding large
compressed rawhide bones upright—formerly held between two
paws—as she chewed. Her back hunched more, neck thicker, stronger. She still jumped to catch toys in midair, ran faster than other
dogs, *as though*, my father would say, *the other leg just got in the way*.

There is beauty in this change, the grace and balance found in
asymmetry. In two creatures from different species of vastly different size using three legs to move through life: her lack, my excess,
this pairing of three.

Wabi sabi, the Japanese aesthetic philosophy closely tied to Zen
Buddhism, insists upon asymmetry and imperfection, aware that
these are signs of life's impermanence and decay. In wabi sabi,
fallen leaves may carry more meaning than those still on the tree;
a ceramic bowl is more beautiful by its lack of uniformity; the com-
position of a painting or photo more deeply felt through its rejection
of centering, the subject somewhere near the frame's edge, amid a
field of blankness. Maybe even a disabled, asymmetrical dog with
her disabled, asymmetrical human can aspire to such beauty.

Wabi sabi expresses a profound love of life through sorrowfully
recognizing its fleeting nature. If there's anything a dog lover knows
and must contend with, it's the fleeting nature of a dog's life, the
speed with which they age and die relative to our own life spans.

Patou and I both became acquainted with life's flux far earlier
than many of our respective species typically do. I shuffled like
my grandmother in my early 20s, periodically experienced uri-
nary incontinence from the age of 17, temporarily lost vision and

needed tinted magnifying lenses in my 30s, and now in my 40s experience cognitive challenges that are more typical of a much older person. In the prime of Patou's life she stopped being able to jump onto furniture, lost her job of pulling me up the stairs, and lost a leg.

Through loss we both gained access to learning what else our bodies could do to persist in this world, how to adapt to the flux and flow of life. Our mobility changes became, for us, the norm. I marvel at the ease with which some people run staircases, as though they're from outer space, but whenever I spot another tri-paw dog's movement, a curtain of serene familiarity washes over me. When Patou and I first approached the sliding glass doors of a pet supply store, each on three legs, I caught sight of our reflection and thought, they're bound to think I'm using my dog to panhandle. I soon came to simply trust and love what I saw in the glass: persistence, trust, grace.

Patou's movement: unmistakable jazz waltz brushes. My movement: the cane's bold stomp followed by a soft hitching shuffle. This music must be wholeness.

After her amputation, Patou continued to live cancer-free for nearly four years. When the same cancer returned in the remaining front leg, its growth was slow, and we treated it with palliative radiation. She began to fall, her front paw flopping and buckling under, resembling the MS symptom "foot drop." I saw the dog's falls through my own experience, and wondered if physical therapy could help her as it had helped me strengthen my leg and relearn, for a while, how to walk. The veterinary physical therapist exercised Patou in water and supplied us with mobility aids: a set of wheels preceded by a string of successive neoprene leg braces to prevent falls, and a harness with long looped handles to support the dog's front end as she descended stairs.

This dog, who carried me up so many flights, welcomed my hand raising her by those handles, lifting her chest to lighten her descent as I braced against the stair rail. A kind of wholeness through asymmetry and time, the tension between impermanence and ongoingness.

Patou's new wheels were more like a rolling walker than a wheelchair; the wheels helped her exercise while supporting her chest's weight. We started using them on quiet sidewalks until she was ready for short jaunts with her wheels at the jogging track of a local park. One day, rounding a turn, we spotted a man using a wheelchair heading toward us. Patou saw him, too, launched into a flat-out run, and rushed straight for him, nearly pulling the leash out of my hand. The man broke into a broad smile and laughed, "No shame in the game, no shame in the game." The beauty of this moment, which I have yet to comprehend fully, was not lost on me: All creatures who persist are whole.

VII

FAMILY

Passing My Disability On to My Children

SHEILA BLACK

WHEN I WAS PREGNANT WITH MY FIRST CHILD, MY OB/GYN referred me to a genetic counselor "just in case."

I have a condition called X-linked hypophosphatemia, or XLH, which results in a form of dwarfism. I was a spontaneous case; there had been no history of XLH in my family before me. No road map.

The counselor did not seem too worried. "Don't sweat it," he said. "Frankly, this is so rare, you'd have to marry a guy from the rickets clinic to pass it on." I gave birth to my first child—my daughter Annabelle—seven months later. She did not have XLH.

Six years later, I stood in a neonatal intensive care unit looking down at my son, Walker. Because my husband and I had a rare blood incompatibility, he needed multiple transfusions. But what I was staring at as he lay in his incubator were his legs—something in them I recognized, a kind of curvature that felt as familiar to me as my own face.

"He has XLH," I said to his doctor. She said, "I wouldn't worry about that—we have enough here to worry about," but a day later she found me in the hall. "You were right," she said. "His phosphorus is very low. We're pretty sure he has what you have."

Because of a mutation on the PHEX gene, people with XLH don't absorb phosphorus, resulting in short stature, bowed legs, soft bones and weak teeth. When I saw the genetic counselor before Annabelle was born, the genetics of my rare condition had not yet been mapped, and in fact, the counselor was wrong. I have a 50 percent chance of passing XLH on. And since the birth of my son, Walker, I've had another daughter, Eliza, who has XLH as well.

Several years ago, a relative of mine, who is quite religious in a way I am not, called me on the phone unexpectedly. She said she wanted to apologize because she had always thought that I should never have children; "God would not want you to have children" is how she put it. Yet now that I did have three of them—three "beautiful children," she'd said—she wanted to let me know she had been wrong. It was a bit of an awkward moment, like when someone tells you that you look fabulous in a way that lets you know how terrible they thought you looked before.

When I found out Walker had XLH, I mourned briefly—mostly for the image I'd had of a tall, gangly teenager, the kind I had never been. But I never once regretted him or his XLH, and I certainly never imagined other people thinking about it or judging me for having had a child with a disability. Her words irked me, but eventually I understood that for an abled person—a person who considers herself "normal"—it is probably difficult to imagine taking the risk of passing on what is considered by most to be a fairly significant disability.

XLH patients, the Merck Manual of Diagnosis and Therapy tells us, are often quite robust apart from their short stature and odd side-to-side gait, and also the pain they suffer—muscle aches, bone aches, "quick to fatigue if asked to walk any distance." My two younger kids and I all hover around five feet. This is not such a big deal for me and my daughter; it is more for my son, and all of us struggle to stand or walk for any length of time.

Occasionally, I come across the term "designer baby," and I am reminded that some parents now have the option to screen or modify the genes of their unborn children to ensure or avoid certain traits. It always gives me a feeling of unease. Obviously, I did not take this route—partly because, at least with my son, I never had to actually make the decision. My third child, Eliza, was a late midlife accident. I chose to have her despite the possibility she would have XLH, but would I have made the same decision in a planned pregnancy or if given a choice much earlier in the process? I can't help suspecting that because of advances in genetic mapping, genetic testing, the sheer range of prenatal choices, chances are that in a generation or two, there will be no one in the world who has XLH, no one who looks like me or my children—at least not in the so-called developed world—and I don't know how to feel about that.

I am aware that some studies do show that short people score less points on "happiness scales," whatever they may mean, but we are not the average study subjects. We are ourselves, individuals; we are what we are—short and proud of it. We are people with a disability.

Sometimes people stop us and ask us what is wrong with us; most of the time I can see that people notice, but they don't say anything. Walker is more visibly disabled, which makes Eliza feel bad. She says sometimes she feels like a fraud because she has the same thing, but in her case "you almost can't tell." Walker rides a bicycle. Eliza does yoga. Both of them pursue these physical activities with fierce and single-minded passion. Both do so because there are other physical activities—walking, running—that they cannot pursue without difficulty. (Oddly, my least athletic child is my oldest, Annabelle, who regularly proclaims she hates all sports.)

Pain—both physical and psychic—is a part of my two younger kids' daily experience, and it is the part that is hardest for me to get over. Perhaps this is what my relative meant. Perhaps sparing your loved one that psychic pain is the reason some people give their short-statured but otherwise perfectly healthy children human growth hormone, so they may grow just a few inches taller.

Most of the time I believe my children will transcend the parts of their disability that might make them suffer. Walker may be only five feet tall, but he is in every conceivable way an engaging personality. He has friends, wild schemes for the future, a wicked, deadpan sense of humor. Eliza is all darting motion—ups and downs. She sings in the shower; does cartwheels on the lawn. She also struggles with an eating disorder and anxiety. And Walker, normally even-keeled, occasionally gives in to fits of rage and frustration when, tired of the effort of simply moving through a day, or being left out at school, he punches walls, rides his bicycle too fast.

How much of this can I really blame XLH for? My oldest, Annabelle, would not say she has a perfect life. At 23, she is floundering a little—unsure what to do with her life or how. She adopts stray dogs. She gets tattoos. She works in a supermarket bakery and is struggling to finish college. She writes killer poems that are also very angsty.

Sure XLH has a cost, but so does life.

I know what the "designer baby" people would say: The more "advantages"—beauty, height, intelligence—the better the life chances, the better the life. But I am not sure I believe them.

Life is more than that.

Of course, I worry about Walker and Eliza. At the same time, I experience so keenly their blazing necessity, their utter beauty. Once I was walking along between them, and I realized all three of us possessed the same awkward-to-most-people "disabled" way of walking. The rush of identification I felt was almost triumphant. *We don't move like other people*, I thought, and *who is to say there are not things we have learned uniquely from our way of moving or being?*

When I was a child in the 1960s, I used to hear or overhear dire predictions about what kind of life I would lead because of my XLH. One teacher in my Catholic primary school said perhaps I should consider becoming a nun because I probably wouldn't marry. A friend of my father's encouraged me to go into biology because "girls who aren't so pretty can still have a pretty terrific career in the sciences." None of these dire predictions came true. I came to think of them as the empty curses of bad fairies; I was blessed, and cursed, to have in most ways an ordinary life.

As a young woman, I had an active sex life (something I'm sure people thought I wouldn't have, but did not say). I had a few bad relationships, a few good ones.

Naturally, I wish better for my children—no psycho ex-boyfriends, no long-term affairs with nicotine or tequila, less time spent worrying about being cool, and more developing their inner resources. But I won't be surprised if they make the same sorts of errors I did. XLH, or any disability, has a lot less to do with all of this than it might appear.

When I asked my children how they felt about the XLH I had passed on to them, both of them spoke of the disability as almost, though not quite, a gift. "It has made me not fit in," Eliza said, "but it has taught me empathy."

"I am sometimes bitter about being so short," Walker said, "and about the pain, but I am very glad to be alive."

I Have Diabetes. Am I
to Blame?

RIVERS SOLOMON

Y FINGERTIPS ARE BRUISED AND POLKA-DOTTED BLACK BECAUSE I am, yet again, getting back on track. A three-month bender of unbridled carbohydrate ingestion has left me a skinsack. I am made of headaches, nausea, vomiting and fatigue. After 10, 12 hours of sleep, I still need a nap because I awake hourly in the night, alternating between trips to the kitchen to guzzle diet soda, iced tea or water and trips to the restroom to urinate it all out.

I swear that this time discipline, grit and force of will—three qualities that have always seemed elusive—will reign. The glucose meter will be my new clock. My life will revolve around its numerical output. After every meal or snack, I will punch a button on the pager-size meter, setting a brief click-clack of machinery in motion before a lancet thrusts into my toughened skin. Because my fingertips have become calloused from years of this, it will sometimes take several pricks before the lancet draws enough blood to register.

Though I've done this thousands of times, I still wince at every jab. I think of medical leeches. I think of bloodletting. It is strange to live in a world where making oneself bleed is the first step to healing.

My sugar-thickened blood reminds me of unrefined petroleum. Lost in one of my many delusions, I wonder if I'm not a human but a gummed-up robot—the model discontinued because its body couldn't understand the most basic and necessary of processes: converting food into fuel.

Soon I will resume the ritual of multiple daily stabbings. I will make a shopping list full of foods I'm not particularly fond of. I'll design a workout plan to accommodate my increasingly troublesome left knee. I'll swallow pills that make my stomach and bowels spasm. I will inject insulin.

I've been diabetic for about 6 years, since age 22. Type 2, I have to add. I am young but fat, so people wonder if I have the sort of diabetes that *just happens* for no reason, typically to very young people, or if I have the sort that I brought on myself through what people perceive as a lack of willpower and self-control.

Culturally, this disease straddles the line between malignant and benign. On the one side, there's the obvious suffering—amputation, heart disease, blindness—side effects of constantly inflamed blood vessels. On the other, there's *just diet and exercise, that's all it takes*, and oral drugs and insulin. There's *you seem fine*. There's the invisibility of the deeply dedicated management it requires.

Diabetes mellitus is a class of metabolic conditions characterized by high blood sugar. The hormone insulin is the vehicle by which sugar—that much disparaged substance—enters our cells from the blood. In Type 1 diabetes, the pancreas no longer produces insulin, which means that sugar has no means to enter cells. In Type 2 diabetes, insulin resistance means that even though insulin is being produced, cells do not respond to it.

While the causes are not completely understood, some combination of genetic predisposition and environmental factors including diet, exercise and stress causes the cells to need more and more insulin to be able to take up sugar from the blood. Weight and diet play a part in developing diabetes Type 2, but genetics is also a factor. As with most diseases and disorders, diabetes has a cascading effect on the body.

Every chronic illness, disease and disability carries with it misunderstandings. Too often society paints disability as a personal failing. A person with chronic pain in her legs, who is not paralyzed but chooses to use a wheelchair, may be seen as weak or lazy.

I've found my fatness compounds this phenomenon. My body is visibly off kilter, a symbol for lethargy, lack of self-regulation, ill health, indolence. Combine this with the misbelief that there is a cure for diabetes—that cure being willpower—and everyone is suddenly an expert on how to fix me. It'd be impossible not to internalize that I am to blame. There is the issue of my blackness, too, which many, because of unconscious bias, interpret as inherently lazy, deviant, sick, unclean.

I've always known my body needed transforming—or that other people thought it did. I was teased and rejected for my body throughout my years in school. I wasn't fat as a child, but I was big. Extraordinarily tall for my age (4-foot-11 in the first grade) and broad-shouldered, I might have excelled at contact sports but I wasn't built for the ballet I longed to do. I saw the attention my grandmother lavished on my skinny cousin contrasted against the frustration she expressed shopping for clothes that fit me. My mother was thankfully kind and nonjudgmental, but when I visited my father over the summers, he put me on grueling diets, including one where I couldn't eat solid foods before midday.

I had started dieting at the age of 6. My mother briefly explained calories to me because it had come up in an unrelated conversation. The next time I ate a slice of bread, I immediately got on our family treadmill until the number on the monitor denoting calories burned matched the number of calories per slice on the package. In later years, I'd secretly drink sample bottles of perfume to try to make myself vomit.

Today, when I do manage to control my diabetes, it's at the cost of almost every other element of my life. Every bite I ingest requires a complex algorithm, calculating ratios of carb to fat to sugar to insulin to the amount of walking I've done. Even when my math is perfect, my sugars rebel. I often fall into dangerous lows (a side effect of taking too much insulin, which sends blood sugar plummeting). I eat an apple to bring my sugar up, and suddenly it's too high again.

Low-carbohydrate diets barely work for me. Even the sugar in a serving of broccoli sends my sugars to uncomfortable highs. I get anxious at parties, at restaurants out with family. Meat, potentially one of the diabetic's safest foods, is often slathered in sugary barbecue sauce or honey glaze.

I weep into my partner's arms when I realize that this level of control is not sustainable. She's been with me since I first got the diagnosis, and after the grief passed, she asked me, "What do you need me to do?" I know she's concerned about my longevity, but she doesn't put that concern before my need for a companion who's not overly invested in my every food choice.

Her gentle support isn't always enough. Diabetes demands perfection, and I am the most imperfect person I know. When eating becomes this exhausting, I simply refrain from food altogether. There is no more surefire way to blood-glucose control than starvation, and I've gone months eating only a small bowl of chicken soup a day, had doctors praise my impressive management.

The extremism with which I tackle diabetes management is directly related to the extremism I apply to food in general. A lifetime of dieting, a lifetime of being told my body is wrong, takes its toll, and I can't help conflating the messages that I am better off starved than fat. Maybe if I could let go of the shame, or more important, if the media, doctors, friends, family could stop shaming me, managing my diabetes wouldn't be this roulette wheel of self-torture. Maybe then, I could finally let go and heal.

10 Things My Chronic Illness Taught My Children

PAULA M. FITZGIBBONS

M Y CHILDREN HAVE A MOTHER WITH A CHRONIC ILLNESS. THEY LIVE with my rheumatoid arthritis just as much as I do. I was given my diagnosis when all three of them were young, and since then I've spent a lot of time worrying about what the daily uncertainty of my condition would mean to them, and whether it would affect their development.

They are all teenagers now, one getting ready for college, and I can attest that my illness has indeed affected them. Here's how.

1. They have acquired patience.

We have spent a lot of time in doctors' offices and hospitals. They've used that time to read, draw, play games and get to know the front-office staff. Sometimes they just watch people or day-dream. At home, I have not always been physically swift in meeting needs or ferrying them to their destinations. Instead of making futile attempts to rush me, they have learned to use the delays to their advantage. My son, for example, has taught himself to play piano during the time it takes me to get moving and ready in the morning. In an age when electronics can fool us into thinking we needn't wait for anything, the patience they've developed is a virtue that would have been otherwise hard to teach.

2. They have developed flexibility.

My children and I have embarked upon many a bike ride or hike, only to have it thwarted by a sudden rheumatic flare. Sometimes we are able to alter the activity to accommodate my pain level. Sometimes we have to scrap the activity altogether. Doing so can be frustrating for my kids. Still, they generally recognize the futility in fretting over the changes—given that the circumstances are beyond our control—and go with the flow. In doing so, they have learned to adapt to sudden changes in plans and problem-solve ways to salvage activities.

3. They have learned to be self-sufficient.

I am not always able to complete household chores. My family would rather I expend my healthy energy on quality togetherness anyway. So while I do what I can of the housework, they pick up the slack. They have been doing everything from their own laundry to keeping the house clean to pet care for so many years that these tasks are natural components of their teenage years. Interestingly, as they have assumed more responsibility, they have also requested more. They often fix entire family meals, barring adults from the kitchen, and serve them with flair. They delight in fixing things around the house, taking pride in our home. Their future roommates and partners will be very thankful for this lesson.

4. They have learned to be considerate.

Autoimmune diseases are unpredictable. There are days when I am unsteady on my feet. This means nobody can leave anything on the floor, lest I trip. There are days when opening a door is a challenge. My children notice such moments and jump ahead to help. Conversely, they notice when I am capable of doing things myself and give me the space to do so. In learning to navigate my illness-related needs, they have developed a sense for when people need help and when they desire independence.

5. They have witnessed commitment in action.

When my rheumatoid arthritis hit, my relationship with my husband changed. As we worked to develop a new normal, he willingly chose to become the de facto caregiver to me while still parenting our three young children. In turn, I had to learn to let go of control and to accept new divisions of labor. We both have had to maintain a healthy sense of humor. Over the years, we have discerned how to tweak our relationship according to my abilities, learning when to be spontaneous (during periods of health) and when to scale back on activities and stress (during flares). Through it all, he has massaged my feet and legs every single night to reduce my pain.

Many kids are grown and out of the house before their parents face health challenges. They don't always see the daily minutiae of caring for one another. A lesson like this can be truly life-changing for young people as they develop a sense of their own future long-term relationships. Rather than falling into a mind-set that youth and perfection are priorities in a relationship, my children have seen firsthand that commitment involves adapting to changing circumstances with a heavy dose of mutual respect.

6. They have developed compassion.

Rheumatoid arthritis can cause pain, swelling, depression, anxiety, fatigue and a slew of other unpleasant symptoms. My children have accompanied me through them all. In doing so, their capacity for compassion has increased exponentially. When they encounter people with their own challenges, they are adept at sensing how they might be present for them if necessary. My eldest daughter has even channeled her compassion into working toward a career as a nurse practitioner.

7. They have learned not to judge by appearances or jump to conclusions.

Having seen me lose the use of my knee in the middle of an ordinary moment, without provocation, my children understand that what they see might not tell a whole story. So when the checker at the market is frowning and seems unfriendly or when an elderly person seems to scowl at them, they are less likely to judge them or take it personally. They recognize that they cannot make assumptions based upon the small amount of information they have.

8. *They have developed an appreciation for service.*

I often hear people speak of service as if it were a box they need to check off at some point, for a transcript or to boost a future career, or an unspoken requirement of their faith. As people living with someone who needs regular help, my children enjoy service without any agenda—except perhaps the intrinsic reward of knowing they were helpful. In turn, I work to serve their needs in ways that I can. With that, they have also learned that all service does not look the same.

9. *They have learned that abilities do not define a person.*

While I'm not always able to kick the ball around or boogie-board with the kids like their father does, I am the choice for a good story, a clever idea, problem solving or a hearty laugh. We all have our thing. This one is simple. I see them working to translate it to their own abilities as well: Just because one sibling can do something doesn't mean they all should master that skill.

Most important, they have learned that their mother is no less a woman, no less interesting, no less a person than I was when I could bike 30 miles with them. This means our relationship is rooted in so much more than what I can do for them.

10. *They have learned that it is OK to experience pain and express strong emotions.*

Both of my daughters also struggle with pain, my eldest from a childhood illness and my youngest from recently diagnosed juvenile rheumatoid arthritis. My eldest child often pushed through her pain to the point of overdoing it. It can be healthy to push through some pain when possible. But at some point she had learned to keep her pain to herself, so much so that on her worst day, I found her sobbing alone in pain.

Since she has seen me with no choice but to wave the white flag to pain at times, she has learned to do the same. All three of us work to maintain balance—knowing when we need to flex and when we need to release, when to put pain first and when to let it fade into the moment.

Though my children would certainly prefer not to have to deal with their mom's having a chronic illness, there have been many gifts along this road. The growth they have experienced and the lessons they have learned are sticking, and for that, we are all grateful.

The Importance of
Finding Family

ALAINA LEARY

M Y MOM AND I HAD ROUTINES. WE WALKED EVERYWHERE—TO THE grocery store, to the bus stop for doctor's appointments and to visit family, and to my school each morning. My favorites were our walks through Lincoln Commons, commonly referred to as Lincoln Park, in our hometown, Malden, Mass., where we'd sit and tell stories underneath our favorite tree.

Before it became a park, Lincoln was the site of an elementary school. A tree had grown inside the school, and the city was planning to demolish the building along with the tree until environmental activists fought to save it. The school was torn down carefully to preserve the tree, and the park was built around it.

Our walks were short, often truncated by pauses, because my mom had Ehlers-Danlos syndrome, a connective tissue disorder that often causes breaks, dislocations and other injuries, and can also cause chronic pain and difficulty walking and standing. Our life was built around my mom's disabilities; she also had a visual impairment, which was why she couldn't drive and we walked everywhere.

It wasn't long before we learned that I am also disabled, inheriting some of my conditions from my mom. When I couldn't walk along a balance beam in preschool, my mom started getting medical professionals involved. She became my biggest disability advocate and champion, getting me set up with school support services, occupational and physical therapy, and a therapist I could talk to about the difficulties of being a disabled kid.

Like every other child, I asked questions: "Why can't you drive a car?" "Will I be able to drive?" "How come I have trouble walking up the stairs and my best friend doesn't?" My mom helped me navigate the early years smoothly, and even when we didn't have all the answers—audiologists were continually confused about my trouble understanding speech, which we later learned was a sensory processing disorder, because I passed every hearing test easily—my mom figured out how to accommodate my needs. We didn't know at first exactly why I had trouble walking up the stairs, but my mom was happy to hold my arm as I ascended each step two feet at a time so that I wouldn't fall.

She was my first role model for what a disabled adult looks like. We didn't use the words "accessibility" and "accommodations," but I learned what they were from firsthand experience. We took public transportation everywhere, and when we occasionally needed to go off the grid, my grandparents and my aunt stepped in as chauffeurs.

My mom didn't do a lot of cooking that required standing for long periods of time, so my childhood was marked by our easy sit-down meals and occasional takeout—and subsequent arguments about whether to get Chinese food or Nana's pizza. When we went outside in the winter, she had to bundle up because of complications from Raynaud's phenomenon, and usually had to dart back into the house to warm up every 10 minutes or so. Most important, she was living proof that disabled adults exist and that they live life just like nondisabled adults do, even if it means doing certain things a little differently.

After my mom died, when I was 11, I didn't just lose my best friend. I also lost my first disabled role model, someone whom I could turn to for advice as I got older about dating, college, work and living on my own with a disability.

I could ask adults about choosing a college, how to advance in a

career and what to look for in my first apartment, but my nondisabled mentors didn't have to think about accessibility or accommodations, or the havoc that a constant physical hustle and lack of
sleep can wreak on my body.

After my mom's death, my dad helped me navigate my severe
digestive issues, which I inherited from him. Luckily, I met other
role models who could help me along the way.

As a senior in college, my career-prep professor, Leah, who has
chronic fatigue syndrome, understood the concerns and fears I had
about my post-grad life. She was happy to guide me through concerns about balancing school, work and health; helped me with
my applications to graduate school; and asked me necessary questions about my course load, accessible housing near campus and
how easy the commute would be for me.

In graduate school I met Lissa, a professor in my graduate program who has multiple sclerosis. I have asked her questions I couldn't
ask most professors about how to excel in my career with a disability.

Just as in the LGBTQ community, which I'm also a part of as
a queer woman, finding camaraderie with other disabled people
means creating a system of found family, people tied together by
their identities and experiences. For those who don't have the good
fortune of a support system, there are mentorship programs.

Nonprofit organizations like the Autistic Self Advocacy Network serve as a way for disabled people to meet one another; the
Youth Leadership Forum is a mentorship program in Massachusetts and other states. There are national and local opportunities
for mentorship, for specific conditions and for disability generally.
Conferences and other events, like the Abilities Expo, are also
places to find disabled community. At Westfield State University
in Massachusetts, where I went for my bachelor's degree, we had
a social support group for students with disabilities. I chose not
to opt in—but I found a vast majority of my friends in this social
circle anyway and wound up creating a found family of disabled
people on campus.

That sense of found family was important not only for maintaining my disability pride, which became harder to hold onto after I lost my mom as a major role model, but also for questions I have about my life.

It is critical for disabled people to find a sense of community. Disability is the only marginalized identity that anyone can enter at any time; one in 20 Americans is disabled, but we're often so disenfranchised that our rights are an afterthought (the Americans With Disabilities Act became law only in 1990). Our strength comes from the relationships with other disabled people that we create, whether these are online or in person, and the lifelong mentorship that these relationships foster.

My mom was the first disabled adult in my life, but not the last. She taught me that I'm strong and capable, like a tree that grew inside an elementary school and demanded to become a part of the world. Everyone should be so lucky. And with the right guidance and access to others willing to help, many people with disabilities can.

Trying to Embrace a "Cure"

SHEILA BLACK

LATELY, THE ONLINE PATIENT SUPPORT GROUP I AM PART OF, THE XLH Network—short for X-linked hypophosphatemia, the genetic illness I and two of my children share—has been blowing up with news of a soon-to-be-released treatment that could very well amount to a cure.

KRN23 is a recombinant antibody that restricts excessive production of a hormone that prevents people with XLH from absorbing phosphorus, leading to our short stature, crooked legs, poor teeth and other symptoms of our type of dwarfism. Ultragenyx, the company responsible for KRN23, has carried out adult tests with no ill effect. Pediatric tests are still underway, but this looks like the real deal. This could truly be a cure. It is hard to explain to anyone who does not have a condition like mine why this feels so bittersweet. But it does.

When Eliza, my youngest child, was born, she was in a neonatal intensive care unit in Albuquerque for three weeks—not because of XLH, but because my husband and I also possess a rare blood incompatibility. My son, born 18 months before, required three exchange transfusions after birth. My daughter, who was as close to a miracle baby as you can possibly imagine, was expected to need the same, but didn't.

While I hung about in that strange suspended animation that is life in the N.I.C.U.—baby girl in an incubator undergoing light therapy, days and nights blurring into one another—one of the doctors, who had taken an interest in the fact that I had a child with *two* rare conditions, said I might want to go hear a lecture taking place that afternoon. It was a presentation on the dialogue between LPs, or Little People (as most people with dwarfism prefer to be called), and the researchers who had developed the prenatal genetic test for achondroplasiac dwarfism, the results of which would obviously be used to allow families to decide whether or not to go ahead and have a child with the condition.

I wish I could remember more of what I saw and heard that day. I sat in the back of a midsize hospital auditorium and listened to doctors and scientists and a representative from Little People of America talk along a bank of microphones. The sound was crackly and hard to hear. There was a PowerPoint presentation and slides of neighborhoods where LPs had lived and grainy pictures of carnivals and circuses where LP families had appeared in the 1930s and 40s. They played video clips of people with achondroplasia who spoke of a strange subversive anguish: Yes, a genetic disorder was being eliminated, and that was a good thing. But at the same time, their world, their culture, was also being erased.

XLH is rare enough that I was well into adulthood before I met anyone with my condition. I was contacted by an early incarnation of the XLH Network. We arranged to meet in a big cavernous restaurant in a strip mall just outside Baltimore. I remember we ordered Caesar salads and large goblets of iced tea, and then someone ordered a glass of wine, and the rest of us did, too. We spoke of our lives, our careers. Some like me had chosen to have children; others had not. One woman I became quite close to, Elaine—a scientist by training—said she could not imagine having children because she felt she and her sister, who also had it, had suffered too much. She was a generation older than me and had not been given vitamin D2 as I had, so she stood about 4 feet 6 inches to my almost five feet. She laughed and said, "Even this makes a difference, and I can tell you my fashion statement is long skirts whatever the occasion."

I don't know that you could make an argument that we, as a

group, have much of a culture in common, but we have had so many similar experiences. Most of us wore braces, spent our childhoods in and out of orthopedic units and had bone surgeries. We had learned that looks *do* matter to the world, even, or maybe especially, when people swear they don't. Yet we had also had sweet, complicated and often triumphant lives. Meeting other people with XLH, I experienced a bond that was nearly primal and hard to explain. The one and only time my family and I encountered another family with XLH outside my support group—in a random encounter in a local Target store—we recognized each other as fellow XLHers instantly and proudly, and left each other in a flurry of high fives.

Lately, I find myself recalling when my children were small, and how XLH was so woven into our lives: dispensing their medicine many times a day, going from the small town where we lived in southern New Mexico to see the specialist in Albuquerque, and mostly the pep talks we all gave one another about how XLH would not stop us from being anything in the world we might want to be, how we knew people thought we looked weird and sometimes treated us badly because of it, but those people were wrong.

By all this I do not mean to say that the prospect of a cure for XLH is a bad thing, only that for people like me, it is a complex one. Certainly, the potential benefits to both individuals and society are real: less struggle and suffering for individuals and families, especially those not financially and socially equipped to overcome them, and perhaps the chance to direct medical attention and limited resources to more life-threatening and debilitating conditions.

But that does not change the fact that to be human often entails finding ways to make what appears a disadvantage a point of strength or pride. XLH does not shorten life-span. It makes walking difficult, and we XLHers suffer more aches and pains than most people. We also look different. When I was a child, this was the main reason I longed for a cure—so I could look like everyone else. Now it is the part of my XLH I cling to a little stubbornly, why I hesitate and wonder: Who would I be without my XLH? Who would my children be?

These are not questions I know how to answer, but I do know that the ambiguous feelings I've been having as the progression toward an XLH cure plays out on my patient listserv stem from issues many more people will grapple with in coming years. My son, Walker, an XLH patient, who is now in engineering school, keeps sending me articles about Crispr, the new gene splicing technology that allows researchers to snip and move even the smallest lines of genetic code, potentially allowing them to correct the smallest genetic anomaly. Recently, the novelist Kazuo Ishiguro commented on Crispr in The Guardian: "We're going into a territory where a lot of the ways in which we have organized our societies will suddenly look a bit redundant. In liberal democracies, we have this idea that human beings are basically equal in some very fundamental way. We're coming close to the point where we can, objectively in some sense, create people who are superior to others."

What is a superior person? What might be lost in the rush toward creating one? It is highly unlikely we will put such technology away, but how do we ensure it does not create the kind of monstrous world H. G. Wells described in "The Time Machine"?

It appears that XLH will be a thing of the past in a few short years. It seems quixotic, or even perverse, to mourn it, but how will we address genetic differences in the future? I can't predict where Crispr and the like will lead, but I do know that ethics and lived experience must be important guides, and that the very knowledge contained in the disability community is perhaps the best place to start, for who better to consider such questions than those of us who have lived with being different?

In My Mother's Eyes, and Mine

CATHERINE KUDLICK

I WAS BLINDFOLDED. MY LEGS DANGLED OFF A CHAIRLIFT HIGH ABOVE THE Colorado ski slope. I nervously licked at little bits of snow that tickled my lips. I was 43, and this was my first time downhill skiing. Whenever the contraption shuddered and bumped, I was convinced that we had become unhitched from the cable and were about to plunge to our deaths.

But assuming my experienced guide was right and we survived the ascent, what then? What should I do with the poles at the top? What if my skis got tangled up? What if the chair knocked me unconscious after I'd dismounted? And how would I explain this to my mother?

I recalled the day not long before when I first broached the topic of my coming training at the Colorado Center for the Blind in Littleton. Hoping to appeal to her adventurous and quirky side, I explained that the program was a bit like Outward Bound. For those who had even slight partial vision, as I do, it involved wearing sleep shades as you did activities—including skiing—that most people assumed could be done only by the sighted.

Mom agreed that this training would help my research on the history of blind people. As a social worker who had been active in the League of Women Voters studying inequalities in the juvenile justice system, she approved of my scholarship on marginalized groups. But accepting that her daughter belonged to one of those groups was another matter. After all these years, the idea that I might be blind enough to benefit from the program didn't seem to register.

I was born two months premature and totally blind with cataracts. Then several months later, I startled when my dad used his new camera flash to take a picture of me nestled in a butterfly chair. This wasn't supposed to happen. Realizing that my eyes might actually be functioning, my parents whisked me off for the first of what would be a series of operations that would punctuate my life, initially giving me sight, then improving it, then saving it when it almost disappeared, and later improving it again. These procedures ultimately allowed me to see about 10 percent of what fully sighted people do.

Thrilled that I wasn't completely blind, I grew up as a profoundly visual person who believed in medical miracles. Each surgery brought some new discovery—the flicker of a candle, shiny wrapping paper, our silky black cat asleep on the golden chair. Everything I could see excited me and still does.

But while most people fear blindness because they perceive it as being lost in the dark, I associated it with being thrust into the spotlight. It was easy to pretend that I had decent vision until the taunting began in elementary school. My cataracts left me wearing thick bifocal glasses and with a condition called nystagmus, rapid muscle movements that make my wandering eyes carry on a rich life of their own. The more I try to hold them still, the more they move. When I was a kid, a doctor explained that my eyes were "always looking for something better to see."

For me, it wasn't always so poetic. One of the many operations I had as a young adult required the surgeon to carve out a larger hole in both pupils, with the painful consequence that my eyes are permanently dilated, and thus extremely sensitive to light. I have trouble walking outside at night or in crowded, chaotic places such as airports or hotels. When I'm tired or anxious, my visual world essentially disappears. I can use only one eye at a time, which means I lack depth perception, and I'm easily con-

fused by shadows, brick walkways, curbs, steps and changes in
floor texture.

I can't say for certain when shame obscured all the other complex feelings about my poor eyesight; I only know that unless it
involved the miracle in the butterfly chair, we seldom talked about
it at home. Nor did we talk about something even more taboo: my
mother's own eyes, and the idea that I inherited my vision problems from her.

Mom functioned through most of her life with one poorly working eye that nobody wanted to admit was rapidly getting worse.
As a child, I somehow never connected the fact that I had the only
mom in all of suburbia who didn't drive with my friends' questions
about why her eyes were different colors. Because Mom didn't wear
glasses and Dad did, I grew up believing that he was the one with
eye problems.

To be fair, we had many enablers to help construct a comfortable, dishonest world. Because blindness induces so much fear in
everyone, friends, teachers, store clerks and even ophthalmologists
colluded to turn my mother and me into people who appeared to
have far better vision. At a young age, I'd memorized the seldom-
changing eye chart so I could perform better on eye exams. I hadn't
set out to deceive anyone; I simply wanted to make people happy
because they acted so pleased when I improved.

So when I'd told her about the Colorado Center for the Blind program all these years later, she said: "But, Cath, you never needed a
blind school before. You've even been teaching college!" Then, with
concern in her voice, she asked, "Has something changed, baby?"

I struggled to find words. Yes, things had been changing. But it
wasn't about what my eyes weren't seeing; it was about how I was
coming to see myself. After decades of pretending to be someone
with decent eyesight, I was at last ready to confront this blindness
that always hovered at the edges of my world. Skiing with a blind-
fold was just the beginning.

I'd like to say we were finally able to speak about this freely, but families being families, we never did. I wish we were able to have chided each other for allowing stigma to pull the wool over our eyes (pun intended!) for so many years. We might have bonded over how much work it takes to spend day after day pretending to see the world just like everyone else. We might have even credited our poor eyesight for giving us a fresh perspective on things that fully sighted people take for granted. Imagine swapping stories about how we coped, about absurd situations, about how we made alternative sense of the world!

But, honestly, I didn't need my mother to do this. Growing up before disability rights and with a mother who berated her for being flawed, my mom had perfected her own strategies and blazed her own trail. Surely, she faced self-doubt and pushed past both her own fears and those of others.

She cultivated nonconformity and invented tools to deal with having to give up a career in New York City in order to be a good wife hauling kids and groceries on a bicycle in suburbia.

In the face of such love and courage, who am I to insist she add embracing blindness to the mix?

When at last my ski guide told me the chairlift had reached the top, I was surprisingly calm. I even imagined taking Mom skiing to thank her for the inner strength and audacity that led me to the top of that mountain in the first place.

Then again, she was right there, just as she has been all along.

A Portrait of Intimate Violence

ANNE FINGER

I N A PHOTOGRAPH TAKEN IN THE EARLY 1960S, I'M SITTING ON THE SIDE porch of our rambling Victorian off Hope Street in Providence, Rhode Island, with my parents and three sisters and brother. We'd just come home from Sunday school at the First Unitarian Church. We girls are wearing skirts and crisp white blouses, stockings held in place by garters. (Pantyhose, which will shortly arrive on the scene, will seem liberating.) My father and brother have crew cuts and narrow ties; they wear drip-dry polyester shirts— perhaps in genuine Dacron polyester, more likely, some off-brand: with five kids in the family, we pinched pennies. We are smiling, clean, white, well-fed, well-dressed, cheerful, bright.

I suppose we could have been described with the adjective "typical." Although at the time, when I was in junior high school, I was aware of our differences. My mother worked when few mothers did. Unlike nearly everyone else on Providence's East Side, we were neither Catholic nor Jewish, but Unitarian. And then, of course, there were my braces and crutches: I'd contracted polio shortly before the introduction of the Salk vaccine.

In the photograph, my right leg, the leg always described as "bad," was tucked behind the one called "good." Someone—maybe one of my parents, maybe the neighbor who took the picture— would have, without speaking of it, probably without even thinking much about it, moved my crutches out of the frame. Years later, during the brief period when I walked with nothing more than a cane, but had let go of my shame about my disability, I'd grab my cane and plant it in front of me when my photograph got snapped, a declaration: This is part of me.

Looking at this picture I remember. And the memory convulses me, disturbs my body, as well as my mind. I am lying on my back on the couch in the living room of our house on Larch Street, my father on top of me, his hands around my neck, pressing harder and harder. Another time, it happened in my bed in the loft at our cottage near Moonstone Beach in Rhode Island's South County. In my bedroom of our house in Providence. It: strangulation. It's hard for me to write the word. I want to say something that sounds less extreme, "choking," "throttling."

According to an institute for violence prevention, "Strangulation is an ultimate form of power and control, where the batterer can demonstrate control over the victim's next breath.

It happened because I had been arguing with one of my sisters about what to watch on television. It happened because I had been making my lunch and my father thought I had the burner on the stove turned too high. It happened for reasons I can't remember.

It surely happened, at least in part, because of alcohol. My father drank every night: the after-work, pre-dinner martinis were followed by a post-dinner highball, whiskey and water, freshened and refreshened and refreshened. Years later an old friend of the family will fix his gaze on me and say, "Anne, I used to come over to your house in the evening, and your father would be stumbling and slurring his words." Then my friend said words that surprised me—I suppose because he was male and strong, and because my own fear of my father had always seemed so private, so solitary: "I was terrified of your father when he was drunk."

And, of course, it happened because of my disability.

My oldest sister began her eulogy at my father's memorial service by saying: "It wasn't easy being my father's daughter." But none of my nondisabled siblings faced the physical rage I did.

There's a statistic about violence against disabled children, from the World Health Organization, drawing on two systematic reviews published in the medical journal the *Lancet*: Disabled children are nearly four times as likely to experience violence as their nondisabled peers.

In some way I find comfort in those figures from the world's leading health agency, from a prestigious medical journal. I'm not alone. It didn't happen to me, as my family has often implied, because I was a difficult child—although I'm sure I was a difficult child. There was some alchemical reaction among my disability, my father's alcoholism, the world around us that saw disability as something shameful.

I don't know the roots of my father's violence. I've often wondered what he witnessed as a child: He had a fraught relationship with his own father, and was fiercely protective of his mother. My grandfather slept in the master bedroom in a bed that cannot have been as impossibly vast as it seemed to me as a child, and my grandmother in a narrow bed in a narrow room under the eaves. Was his anger at his own father, his devotion to his mother, a result of violence he'd witnessed? He'd served in the Navy in the Pacific during World War II, and a few times, in a strangely detached manner—it seemed simultaneously joking and bombastic—he'd talked about Japanese soldiers being shot as they tried to surrender. (Years later, someone would recount being gang raped to me in a similar fashion.) Childhood, wartime trauma? I will never know.

My father was also fun, and generous. When I was 6 years old, recovering from surgery with my leg encased in a plastic cast during a sweltering summer, crying with pain as I tried to sleep, my father stood in the doorway, with a broom in his back pocket, dancing until I laughed and finally fell asleep. We rode in his Model A—he'd bought it for 10 dollars from one of his students—down rutted country roads, all seven of us in the car, belting out: "For it's hi-hi-hee in the field artillery. Shout out your numbers loud and strong!" At our beach house, after a dinner of lobsters and steamed clams, he'd join us on the deck as we spit watermelon seeds at each other. An hour or two later, we'd all troop off to the Vanilla Bean for ice cream. After the U.S. invasion of Cambodia in May of 1970, my father made a gigantic kite with a peace symbol on it to fly at his college's graduation (although it turned out to be too large to fit it into his car).

The thing about intimate violence is it's so damn intimate. Not just the closeness of the press of my father's hands around my neck, but the complications of my life and his life, entwined.

Alcoholism, trauma. Still, in the end, I come back to disability:

Did my body somehow read, in all those complicated twists and turns of the inner life of a family, as outer evidence of all that was wrong behind the doors of our home? Did it seem like I was to blame for my disability? After all, my family had been fed the lie that polio could be overcome with enough grit and perseverance. Despite weekly treks to physical therapy, exercises every night after dinner, repeated surgeries, I remained disabled. In that postwar era it seemed that everything was just going to get better and better and better: Cars would have bigger fins, women's skirts would grow fuller and fuller; soon there would be jetpacks and robots doing housework. And there was my body, stubborn, inescapable—in the eyes of the world, bad: something to be rid of.

VIII

JOY

Mishearings

OLIVER SACKS

O NE DAY, WHEN I HEARD MY ASSISTANT KATE SAY TO ME, "I AM GOING to choir practice," I was surprised. I have never, in the 30 years we had worked together, heard her express the slightest interest in singing. But I thought, *who knows? Perhaps this is a part of herself she has kept quiet about; perhaps it is a new interest; perhaps her son is in a choir; perhaps. . . .*

I was fertile with hypotheses, but I did not consider for a moment that I had misheard her. It was only on her return that I found she had been to the *chiropractor.*

A few days later, Kate jokingly said, "I'm off to choir practice." Again I was baffled: *Firecrackers? Why was she talking about firecrackers?*

As my deafness increases, I am more and more prone to mishearing what people say, though this is quite unpredictable; it may happen 20 times, or not at all, in the course of a day. I carefully record these in a little red notebook labeled "PARACUSES"— aberrations in hearing, especially mishearings. I enter what I *hear* (in red) on one page, what was actually *said* (in green) on the opposite page, and (in purple) people's reactions to my mishearings, and the often far-fetched hypotheses I may entertain in an attempt to make sense of what is often essentially nonsensical.

After the publication of Freud's "Psychopathology of Everyday Life" in 1901, such mishearings, along with a range of misreadings, misspeakings, misdoings and slips of the tongue were seen as "Freudian," an expression of deeply repressed feelings and conflicts.

But although there are occasional, unprintable mishearings that make me blush, a vast majority do not admit any simple Freudian interpretation. In almost all of my mishearings, however, there is a similar overall sound, a similar acoustic *gestalt*, linking what is said and what is heard. Syntax is always preserved, but this does not help; mishearings are likely to capsize meaning, to overwhelm it with phonologically similar but meaningless or absurd sound forms, even though the general form of a sentence is preserved.

Lack of clear enunciation, unusual accents or poor electronic transmission can all serve to mislead one's own perceptions. Most mishearings substitute one real word for another, however absurd or out of context, but sometimes the brain comes up with a neologism. When a friend told me on the phone that her child was sick, I misheard "tonsillitis" as "pontillitis," and I was puzzled. Was this some unusual clinical syndrome, an inflammation I had never heard of? It did not occur to me that I had invented a nonexistent word—indeed, a nonexistent condition.

Every mishearing is a novel concoction. The hundredth mishearing is as fresh and as surprising as the first. I am often strangely slow to realize that I *have* misheard, and I may entertain the most far-fetched ideas to explain my mishearings, when it would seem that I should spot them straight away. If a mishearing seems plausible, one may not think that one *has* misheard; it is only if the mishearing is sufficiently implausible, or entirely out of context, that one thinks, "This can't be right," and (perhaps with some embarrassment) asks the speaker to repeat himself, as I often do, or even to spell out the misheard words or phrases.

When Kate spoke of going to choir practice, I accepted this: She *could* have been going to choir practice. But when a friend spoke one day about "a big-time cuttlefish diagnosed with ALS," I felt I must be mishearing. Cephalopods have elaborate nervous systems, it is true, and perhaps, I thought for a split second, a cuttlefish *could* have ALS. But the idea of a "big-time" cuttlefish was ridiculous. (It turned out to be "a big-time publicist diagnosed with ALS.")

While mishearings may seem to be of little special interest, they can cast an unexpected light on the nature of perception—the perception of speech, in particular. What is extraordinary, first, is that they present themselves as clearly articulated words or phrases, not as jumbles of sound. One *mis*hears rather than just *fails* to hear.

Mishearings are not hallucinations, but like hallucinations they utilize the usual pathways of perception and pose as reality—it does not occur to one to question them. But since all of our perceptions must be constructed by the brain, from often meager and ambiguous sensory data, the possibility of error or deception is always present. Indeed, it is a marvel that our perceptions are so often correct, given the rapidity, the near instantaneity, with which they are constructed.

One's surroundings, one's wishes and expectations, conscious and unconscious, can certainly be co-determinants in mishearing, but the real mischief lies at lower levels, in those parts of the brain involved in phonological analysis and decoding. Doing what they can with distorted or deficient signals from our ears, these parts of the brain manage to construct real words or phrases, even if they are absurd.

While I often mishear words, I seldom mishear music: notes, melodies, harmonies, phrasings remain as clear and rich as they have been all my life (though I often mishear *lyrics*). There is clearly something about the way the brain processes music that makes it robust, even in the face of imperfect hearing; and, conversely, something about the nature of spoken language that makes it much more vulnerable to deficiencies or distortions.

Playing or even hearing music (at least traditional scored music) involves not just the analysis of tone and rhythm—it also engages one's procedural memory and emotional centers in the brain; musical pieces are held in memory and allow anticipation.

But speech must be decoded by other systems in the brain as well, including systems for semantic memory and syntax. Speech is open, inventive, improvised; it is rich in ambiguity and meaning. There

is a huge freedom in this, making spoken language almost infinitely flexible and adaptable—but also vulnerable to mishearing.

Was Freud entirely wrong then about slips and mishearings? Of
course not. He advanced fundamental considerations about wishes,
fears, motives and conflicts not present in consciousness, or thrust
out of consciousness, which could color slips of the tongue, mishearings or misreadings. But he was, perhaps, too insistent that
misperceptions are wholly a result of unconscious motivation.

Collecting mishearings over the past few years without any
explicit selection or bias, I am forced to think that Freud underes-
timated the power of neural mechanisms, combined with the open
and unpredictable nature of language, to sabotage meaning, to
generate mishearings that are irrelevant both in terms of context
and of subconscious motivation.

And yet there is often a sort of style or wit—a "dash"—in these
instantaneous inventions; they reflect, to some extent, one's own
interests and experiences, and I rather enjoy them. Only in the
realm of mishearing—at least, my mishearings—can a biography
of cancer become a biography of Cantor (one of my favorite math-
ematicians), tarot cards turn into pteropods, a grocery bag into
a poetry bag, all-or-noneness into oral numbness, a porch into a
Porsche, and mere mention of Christmas Eve a command to "Kiss
my feet!"

Space Travel

A Vision

DANIEL SIMPSON

O NE NIGHT, I HAD A DREAM (OR HALF-DREAM) ABOUT SWINGING ON MY own for the first time. It started out as a kind of interview, as though I were getting help coming up with an idea for a poem. Someone asked me what I was wearing. I said shorts. Then, after thinking a few seconds, I remembered the short-sleeved seer-sucker shirts we used to wear, my twin brother, Dave, and I. I may have been about 4, about the age of the boy I can hear crying in the street as I write this—all those partials in his voice, all that open-mouthed speech, full of longing, you can't quite understand.

My mother was going to push the swing, the wooden kind you often find on a school playground. She pushed a few times, a bump and a jerk every time her hands broke my backward glide. The sun shone. Early spring. Birds. Maybe I had just awakened from a nap, feeling fresh and alive, yet in that semiconscious state of relocating the world. For the first time, I really tried to pull on the chains. I didn't know to kick out with my feet at the same time, or to lean back into the pull. I bounced hard, but adjusted quickly on my next arc. I don't remember anyone telling me to try this, but they probably did. I smoothed out the pull and felt myself going higher.

I'm swinging, I thought.

Such a simple, obvious thought. But it was the first time I'd had it. *I don't need my mother to push now.* She seemed to know it, too, backing away from my higher trajectory. I was free, a blind boy traveling on his own. I could accelerate. I could be daring. No sunroof necessary. The wind rushed at my face, then at my back. It would still be a while before I would buy tickets to get on carnival swings that flew high above loud rock music at a giddy, centrifugal angle. I would not yet need them to be my wings.

I remember visiting the Pealings, long-distance friends of my parents, and going out to a field with their son David to shoot off his model rocket. It was the early 60s, in the shadow of Sputnik, and he was the first kid I knew to have his own launcher. We had a portable tape recorder that we took with us to capture the event. The launch offered little to the blind observer, just a small, albeit exciting, fizz of fire right before the rocket lifted off. After that, it went up noiselessly and landed too far away to hear it come down.

My brother and I had a record, one of those 33–1/3s the size of a children's 78, with sounds from John Glenn's first flight on Friendship 7. We listened to live broadcasts of those early flights at school, usually over the public address system. Those and the World Series were the only events we got to hear in class.

Maybe it seems like nothing special for boys (or girls) to be interested in outer space. But for a person who cannot even see the moon, everything seems even farther away. You might as well be sending something out into another solar system. I just believe there is a moon because my father said there was, and because my grandfather watched it to determine planting times, and because too many love poets talked about it for me to pretend that it was just one or two people's fantasy.

I met a man who had seen the moon all his life and who was probably very worried about the time when he would see it no longer. I was standing at 34th and Walnut, talking to a fellow graduate student about political poetry. So far, it had been a great day: lunch with a friend, a conference with my poetry instructor, a great conversation about Allen Ginsberg and Robert Lowell with another professor, and three hours of reading Stanley Kunitz essays in the library. As soon as my classmate said goodbye and headed for a coffee shop across Walnut, a man who sounded to be in his 30s said to me in a polite and slightly plaintive voice, "Excuse me, sir, but may I have a word with you?"

I said yes, and then his mother took over. "This is Joe," she said, "and Joe is losing his sight. We saw you last week but we didn't get a chance to talk to you. You have a beautiful dog. We admired him (is it him or her?) last week, and Joe has an application . . ."

"Yes, here in my pocket," Joe broke in.

"In his pocket," she continued. "It's from the Seeing Eye. I'm sure that's where you must have gotten your dog." I explained that, no, I went to another guide dog training school and that there were at least a dozen schools of that kind in the United States. But I wanted to turn the conversation to Joe.

He seemed happy to know I had gone to college. "How did you take notes? You surely didn't have someone take them for you, did you?" I told him about the Braille slate and stylus I used then, and about the Braille printer and computers with speech I use now. "How do you get your books?" he asked. And so we talked about that. Maybe five minutes of talking, Joe and me, his mother standing quietly. When she spoke, she burst into tears, "When you have to go to a place, it's nice to know someone who's already been there."

I feel a little melodramatic recording this, but when I stop and think about it, I know it's not. My ears were clogged by a cold. I had been struggling all week to hear traffic accurately as I attempted to cross busy streets. I think that put me even more in sympathy with Joe than I might otherwise have been.

I am an ambassador from a distant land. For Joe, I might as well have come from the moon, which I can't see. I might as well be John Glenn. Except that Joe doesn't have to go to the moon. He only has this other journey in front of him. John Glenn, after lifting off, said everything was "A-OK." I don't know if it was he or Mission Control who followed with, "May the good Lord ride all the way."

When I left Joe, I didn't think to give him my phone number. "May God go with you," he said. "I hope things go well for you, too," I replied, turning to cross 34th. His mother said goodbye in a level voice; she had stopped crying.

I think now of my mother and how she wept when the doctor confirmed that Dave and I had indeed been born blind. I picture her crumpling into the nearest chair the way one sometimes does when bad news knifes through that thin veil of hope mixed with denial. Who were my parents' ambassadors? Who told them that this ride with blind children could be a good ride all the way? I hope Joe is out there somewhere, swinging high above the landscape, the wind whistling in his ears, his mother looking on and beaming.

Learning to Sing Again

ANNE KAIER

ONE SUMMER AFTERNOON NOT LONG AGO, ALONE IN A MEDIEVAL CHApel in central France, I began to sing. Tentatively at first, testing the acoustics, as well as my voice, which, after 71 years of use, wavers in song. Would it reverberate pleasingly against the ancient stone?

It did. I relaxed my throat and sang louder, steadying the soprano notes of a Vivaldi fugue as they rose on a column of air and thrummed through my slightly scaly lips. I sang fully conscious of the pure physical joy of it—a pleasure beyond the flowing endorphins that singing releases. I tightened my abdominal muscles to support deeper breaths and marveled at the sound that vibrated in my vocal cords and finally resounded in the chambers of my skull. For me, this was a late-blooming pleasure. Over the years I had retreated from my body. I did not believe it could make beauty or give delight.

I have lamellar ichthyosis, a genetic skin disorder that manifests in dry scaling. My skin peels perpetually and my face is abnormally red. For many years, I coped with my body by divorcing my mind from it. Denial can be a useful strategy—it has helped me get up in the morning, ignore the persistent itching and walk out into the world each day. But obviously there's a downside: It's hard to feel pleasure in your arms and breasts and lips when you are estranged from them.

Many a wise therapist will encourage people with a disability to find a way to love their own body. Mine has. But we both recognize that because I had neglected mine for so long, I needed to find something beautiful in my body to negotiate terms of endearment with it. Singing ultimately revealed that beauty.

As a child, I sang in church. In fact, families in my small Catholic parish chanted the same melodies—the haunting "Tantum Ergo," for example—that medieval French families sang in Romanesque cathedrals. Standing next to my father, who sang with a musician's poise, I routinely chimed in. At home, we had a Chickering baby grand on which Dad played show tunes every night. I often sat next to him, singing along lustily but imperfectly, thinking that my notes, which came in bursts, would never equal his smooth tenor.

The real damper on my musical instincts arrived in the form of piano practice. Every afternoon in elementary school, I plunked my discordant fingers in the cracks between the keys, not because I didn't know the score, but because the thickened skin on the tips of my fingers prevented me from feeling the ivories—literally.

As a child, I never let myself recognize what was wrong. I just drew back, in my mind, from a body whose imperfections I didn't understand. My parents, deep in denial that my skin problem was anything but a medical matter, didn't recognize how ill-suited for the piano my taut hands were. Finally, when I was about 13, distressed by my bungling, I convinced my mother that it was time to stop. I left the piano bench with relief and a dimly felt regret.

In high school, my musical tendencies suffered another blow. The inexperienced nun who conducted the choir asked me to sing alto, below my natural range. I couldn't drive my voice down to find the low notes; worse, I kept hearing the higher soprano line and so I sang it somewhere in the middle—like a mezzo-soprano would—fine for my body, but not in the score as written. The choir director tried to work with me and warned me that if I didn't improve, I would be asked to leave the group. Increasingly miserable, I finally just mumbled in the back row until the inevitable dismissal. I now had more reason to be ashamed of my clumsiness.

So by age 15, I was convinced that my body could not make

powerful music. I didn't even try to sing again until I was 35 and a friend gave me some smart advice.

One raw spring afternoon, Mary Heiberger and I walked down Spruce Street near the University of Pennsylvania where we worked as career counselors. A musician herself, Mary remarked that I had a pleasant speaking voice and asked me if I sang with a group. We had had this conversation before. I'd always demurred, retelling, with flourishes, my story of being booted out of the high school chorus. But this time she persisted, leaning down toward me as we walked. She must have sensed something brimming in me, some old desire to touch music in an intimate way. My father had recently died, and as heartbreaking as that was, I sensed I might feel freer to open my voice now that I didn't have to compete with his confident tenor.

On the windy street, Mary got practical. "Look," she said, "maybe you're not an alto. Get your voice tested. Take a few lessons." In the coming weeks, I thought about it.

About the same time, I began to see a therapist for the first time. Very gradually, I started to talk about my skin disorder and how it had influenced my life. All my confused and conflicted feelings about my body began to surface.

I began to think more clearly about its flaws and its potential. I certainly didn't come to love my skin in any triumphant way, but as I thought about what my body offered me, I began to mull Mary's advice. Was it possible, I wondered, that I too could sing the choral music I'd loved in medieval chapels in Oxford when I had been a graduate student there? Perhaps. I consulted Mary again; she recommended a teacher.

So one April day I stood before a Steinway grand in a room out of an Edith Wharton novel, with palm trees and overstuffed chairs. I sang "America the Beautiful" twice—once in the lower register and once in the higher. "You are a soprano," the teacher said, decisively, "and you have a big voice."

That changed everything. I took lessons, improved my tone and joined a community choir that performs for the public every winter and spring. At the first rehearsal, I trailed behind the other sopranos. I hadn't sight-read music for 20 years. Nevertheless, I felt exhilarated. *I am singing Beethoven*, I said to myself, even as my back itched as if it were aflame. By the middle of that rehearsal, I felt my lungs expand and notes begin to resonate in the hollows of my head. For a while I merely glanced at this physical pleasure, but as my voice gained power over the weeks of rehearsal, I began to trust my body to do what I asked it to do. I started to feel confident enough to sing fortissimo measures with the full power of my big voice and to enjoy that act profoundly.

In truth, I still cringe sometimes at the sight of my scaly hands and bright red face. But I love singing. With all my flaws as a singer—wrong notes, wavering in the higher octaves as I age, I know that when I am singing at my best I make beauty and feel powerful physical pleasure. I am a singer; my body is my instrument.

Sensations of Sound

On Deafness and Music

RACHEL KOLB

WHEN I GOT A COCHLEAR IMPLANT AT 20, AFTER BEING PRO-
foundly deaf for my entire life, hearing friends and
acquaintances started asking me the same few ques-
tions: Had I heard music yet? Did I like it? What did it sound like?

Aside from the amplified noises I'd heard through my hearing
aids, which sounded more like murmurs distorted by thick insula-
tion swaddling, I had never heard music, not really. But that did
not mean I wasn't in some way musical. I played piano and guitar
as a child, and I remember enjoying the feel of my hands picking
out the piano keys in rhythm, as well as the rich vibrations of the
guitar soundboard against my chest. I would tap out a beat to many
other daily tasks, too.

For several years, I became privately obsessed with marching
in rhythm when walking around the block, counting out my steps
like a metronome: *One, two. One, two.* Watching visual rhythms,
from the flow of water to clapping hands and the rich expression
of sign language, fascinated me. But in the hearing world, those
experiences often didn't count as music. And I gathered that my
inability to hear music, at least in the view the people I knew,
seemed unthinkable.

"So you can't hear the beautiful music right now?" I remember
someone asking me when I was an undergraduate. We sat in a restaurant where, presumably, some ambient melody played in the background. When I said no, she replied, "Wow, that makes me feel sad."

Sad. This is how some hearing people reacted to my imagined lifetime without music. Did it mean that some part of my existence was unalterably sad, too? I resisted this response. My life was already beautiful and rich without music, just different. And even if listening to music did not yet feel like a core part of my identity, I could be curious.

Once I got the cochlear implant, a transmitter of rough-hewn sound that set my skull rattling and my nerves screeching, I found that music jolted my core in ways I could not explain. Deep percussion rhythms burrowed into my brain and pulsed outward. A violin's melody pierced and vibrated in my chest, where it lingered long after the song had ended. Other tunes sounded overburdened, harsh and cacophonic, and I longed to shut them off and return to silence—as I still do.

The new contrast I'd found, between the thrill of sound and the relief of silence, showed me something that I had perhaps known for my entire life, but had never been able to articulate. Music was not just about sound. It never had been. Music, to me, also was, and is, about the body, about what happens when what we call sound escapes its vacuum and creates ripples in the world.

The summer after I got my cochlear implant, I started to explore more of what music might mean to me. I picked out some notes on the piano again. I went to my first symphony concert. That overwhelming time, and all the new things I was hearing, gave me new license to go make music of my own. At the symphony, the cochlear implant whisked me into a flush of sound, but I was still enthralled by the visual—watching the physical artistry of the musicians with their instruments. Not long after, I discovered the art of music videos performed in American Sign Language. The work of talented deaf artists like Jason Listman and Rosa Lee Timm made some songs, which I'd previously listened to with mild interest, suddenly roar to life. I watched those songs in ASL, and that was when I truly *felt* them, in a way an auditory or written rendering could never provide.

Soon after, I tried dancing. It wasn't that I hadn't danced before—just that I'd felt embarrassed. There had been a time, once, when I'd found myself on the dance floor surrounded by hearing friends who belted out song lyrics I couldn't understand. I'd fielded the usual questions from them about how much of it I could *really* hear, which made me ask myself why I was there. Wasn't deaf dancing an oxymoron, after all? Now, as the deaf model Nyle DiMarco has clearly shown on "Dancing With the Stars," the answer is no—but I freely confess that, in the days before his performances, I had to discover this for myself.

Again, my cochlear implant gave me license to try. When a friend persuaded me to go dancing for the first time in years, I discovered that, even though I undeniably enjoyed listening to the music, my favorite songs were the ones that thrummed with a deep rhythm, that sent the bass vibrating through my body. I danced not only by what I heard, but also by what I felt. The physical motion of dancing, once I released myself to it, swirled through my core. Then, when my friend and I started signing along to the lyrics, the realization hit me: *this* celebration of feeling, motion, sensation and language was what mattered when I experienced music.

Not only does music ingrain itself in our bodies in ways beyond simply the auditory, it also becomes more remarkable once it does.

"Can you hear the music?" Even though I now can, I think this question misses the point. Music is also wonderfully and inescapably visual, physical, tactile—and, in these ways, it weaves its rhythms through our lives. I now think a far richer question might be: "What does music *feel like* to you?"

I Dance Because I Can

ALICE SHEPPARD

Y HANDS ARE COLD, CLAMMY. THEY ALWAYS ARE WHEN I'M NER-
vous. And I'm nervous, all right. My heart is pound-
ing, too.

I have about 30 seconds to settle myself before I swing my right
leg up onto the top surface of our ramp stage set, pull hard on the
metal drawer handles that are affixed to its edges, and slide up on
my stomach into the opening position of the dance. I take a deep
breath, close my eyes; the cold surface squeaks as I slide on it. I
count another 45 seconds or so before the music starts.

The dance is called "DESCENT," and it is a creation of the collective Kinetic Light. Over the course of the next hour, I will launch
my body up down and around the curvaceous plywood structure of
our set. Bathed in the stunning projections of our lighting, video
and projection designer, Michael Maag, I will sit on its peak, dive
into its underworld and join my dance partner, Laurel Lawson, as
we move from wheelchair to floor, platform to valley, pushing, pulling, intertwining ourselves until the final moment when together
we leap for the edge.

I was not supposed to be a dancer; I grew up playing music and
dreaming of working in an orchestra. I pivoted at the last minute, studied languages, went to graduate school, became a professor, and never looked back at the arts until I saw the dancer Homer
Avila perform at a conference on disability studies in 2004. We
spoke after the show. At the time, I could not have guessed the
effect his words would have on me. I somewhat tipsily accepted his

dare to take a dance class. I did not know that Homer would soon be dead and that his words would ignite a curiosity that would become a fiery passion for dance. Two years later, I resigned from my academic job and began to train as a dancer.

Even now, nearly 15 years later, people often ask why I dance. I tell them because of the way it feels, because of the pleasure, because I can. Mostly, though, these answers land awkwardly. I see my interlocutor soften. Sometimes, their internal/external filter fails: *Of course, someone with your limitations must get enjoyment from moving; it must feel good, considering; movement probably even helps, right? Therapy?*

None of this is the case. Dance is often more injurious than therapeutic. I do not work from a deficit-based understanding of my body. But it is true that I enjoy it. Immensely. I have fallen in love with stretching, pushing, sweating: with the very effort of moving. I have fallen in love with dancing: its power and freedom are like nothing else I know.

In the studio, I listen carefully, trying to learn what my body teaches. Being on stage is sometimes surreal. For one brief evening, I am connected to several hundred people at once. We are in a conversation that frequently has no words. I cannot see them, but I can feel them. Sometimes, I know we are breathing together.

The dance is in full swing. Twenty minutes into it I slide from my stomach into the seat of my wheelchair. Focused on Laurel, I slip one hand underneath my butt and pull out the strap that secures me to the chair. It makes a deeply satisfying noise as the Velcro unfolds. She flirts; I flirt right back. We are two disabled women investigating what it might mean to build an interracial queer relationship. The act of strapping oneself into a chair is so familiar to those who are or who know wheelchair users. For the select few of us who love a wheelchair user the sound of that Velcro may well recall moments of intimacy. It is such a cultural moment.

Resonant. Political. And, I hope, beautiful. I did not have to tell
Michael how to light this moment. Michael is also a wheelchair
user: he knew. I can feel the way he holds us in his light. It is sexy.
Intimate. He picks up my arm, the strap. Michael is dancing right
there with us.

Of course, nondisabled people appreciate this moment. But
what it actually means to see and feel strapping on stage, to hear
and recognize the sound of Velcro unfurling is different, more
complex for those of us in the disability community. For some,
the choice to strap publicly was controversial—too private or simply to show on stage; for others, it was revelatory, a moment of
celebration. Strapping and intimacy became a regular aspect of
post-show conversations. What does it mean to show a sex scene
that happens out of our chairs? What are the politics of showing
a sex scene in our chairs?

Culturally, the United States is no longer in an "art for art's sake"
moment. Even though we do not always know what change looks
like, we claim meaningful relationships between art and social
justice: particularly, when the artist is from a socially minoritized
or stigmatized group. Art by disabled artists, for example, is seen as
being tied to the artist's own disability status, as overcoming that
status, responding to the tribulations of disabled life. Sometimes,
counter even to the creator's actual focus, the assumed artistic
intent of such work is educating nondisabled people about disability rights, etiquette, and nudging people to think differently about
disability and equity in the world. This is limiting.

Linking art so directly to social change can detrimentally tie
cultural production to broad societal narratives, making it hard
for everyone to understand art outside the lines of those stories.
Culturally specific work like disability art can have meaning in
a number of different realms. As people invested in nuance and
complexity, we owe it to ourselves and the creators of the work to
educate ourselves in the traditions and legacies of the community
so we can appreciate the work outside the narrowness of framings.

"DESCENT" takes place on an architectural, sculptural set that we call the ramp. It is a ramp like no other. Unlike the access ramps that enable wheelchair users to avoid stairs, this ramp is beautiful. It is visually inviting; pushing up its surfaces is a pleasure filled challenge. When we roll down, our hands off our wheels, our chairs turn automatically, spinning either out of control and into the ground or, if we are perfectly balanced, we turn seemingly endlessly. The ramp was designed by 12 students at Olin College for a class co-taught by Sara Hendren and Yevgeniya Zastavker. Under the regulations of the Americans With Disabilities Act, the specifications for an ideal wheelchair access ramp are quite clear, as are the defining parameters of maximum gradient, minimum width, appropriate materials, and so on. The codes make no mention of what it might feel like to use these ramps; they focus on what it takes to enter a building safely. Though perfectly usable and necessary, I see these designs as examples of #rampfail. Disabled people want more than access.

The scholar and activist Simi Linton describes the raw pleasure of rolling down hills in a manual wheelchair. Her words encapsulate the experience of so many ramp users. With support of the college, the Olin students designed for beauty and for the maximum potential of pleasurable wheeled movement. The resulting set reconceptualizes our understanding of what ramps can be; this ramp is art. As Rosemarie Garland-Thomson puts it, the ramp is "aesthetically non-compliant" with the Americans With Disabilities Act.

———

The creaking plywood on the ramp and skidding sounds of our tires on its surface support me as I stretch out my hands to Laurel. Her body pushes into mine with just enough momentum that, hands intertwined, we shoot towards the edge of the ramp. The ramp catches us and carries us over to the other side and then we drift from side to side down the ramp; we are held in Michael's light, the audience breathes softly with us, the music fades, and the sounds of the ramp fill the theater until we can move no more. The ramp exhales into silence; the first half closes as the theater goes dark.

Disability culture and aesthetics are bound up with access, but not in the sense elucidated in the law. We are accustomed to thinking of accessibility as being about an accommodation that bridges the gap between the disabled and nondisabled worlds. But activists like Mia Mingus and disability justice communities like the *Sins Invalid* collective emphasize access as a process and a way of creating connection between disabled people, a way of knowing and being in the world.

Members of the disability community have been involved in all aspects of the show, from preshow communications and trainings, to front of house staffing, to an upcoming seminar. People have flown in from across the country to share in this event. The audience feels like family, and we have done our best to welcome them as opposed to accommodate them—the language used to describe accessibility in the law. We did not get it all right; I know that. But access is also about the commitment to learn and be with each other differently. Next time, we will learn more.

The music crescendos. From the top of the ramp, I watch as Laurel pushes at top speed part way down the slope. She flings herself at the peak. Before I even fully realize it, my chair is in motion. I'm heading toward her; I throw my arms out, land on top of her, and grab the peak. My heart is thudding; Michael flashes the lights; Laurel shifts; we hang there, together.

Stories About Disability Don't Have to Be Sad

MELISSA SHANG

Like any middle schooler, I usually start my day with cereal. Every morning, after brushing my teeth, I have a bowl of Cinnamon Toast Crunch with milk, and try to catch all the flakes with my spoon before they go soggy. I get dressed for the day, and try to put on some makeup before my mom yells at me for hogging the bathroom. Then I go catch the bus.

While in most other ways I'm just your typical eighth grader, I also happen to have been born with Charcot-Marie-Tooth, a form of muscular dystrophy. Charcot-Marie-Tooth is a degenerative nerve disease that causes muscles in my arms and legs to atrophy over time. I wear leg braces and use a wheelchair to get around, and have an aide at school who helps me spin my locker combination. Every morning, an accessible bus arrives at my house to pick me up. Actually, it's more of a van, with a "School Bus" sign on top.

For the most part, despite my wheelchair and knowledge of medical terminology (you build that kind of vocabulary when it's about your own limbs), my daily reality is mostly the same as that of my classmates. I groan over the same math and science homework, giggle with the same friends, and like every other adolescent, I probably spend too much time on my phone. As a girl with a disability, I know that my story is not a sad one.

For the past four years, I've been trying to convince everyone else as well that my story doesn't have to be a sad one. In 2013, I started a Change.org petition asking American Girl, my favorite doll company, to make a doll with a disability. As a longtime fan of the company, whose dolls are accompanied by books and movies with positive stories of girls overcoming challenges, I wanted to see a story with a heroine who was in a wheelchair like me. The petition got 140,000 signatures, and got a lot of news coverage. People clearly wanted to see kids with disabilities featured in upbeat ways.

It would not be fair to say that American Girl completely ignores disability. They do make accessories for dolls like a wheelchair, crutches, a hearing aid and a diabetes care kit. In one of the stories there is a secondary character in a wheelchair; in another, a boy in the hospital with polio, and the 2017 Girl of the Year has a stutter. But these were not the characters I wanted to see.

I was inspired to take matters into my own hands and write a book of my own, starring a girl with a disability. I knew exactly what genre of book I wanted to write. I've never been a fan of "great children's literature" that was somber or tragic. My friends and I have loved the Cupcake Diaries series, paperbacks with pink covers that described four best friends and their adventures together, making cupcakes. Not exactly heavy stuff, but fun to read. I wanted to write something like the Cupcake Diaries, but starring a middle-school girl with a disability and her filmmaking adventures with her best friends. Instead of making cupcakes, they would make special-effect YouTube videos.

My older sister Eva helped me set up a Kickstarter campaign to hire an editor. We wrote the first draft of the book, called "Mia Lee Is Wheeling Through Middle School," and found a literary agent. Using our money from our Kickstarter campaign, we hired someone to help us edit our draft into a polished copy, then sent it out to publishing houses.

When the responses started to come in, they were almost all the same: For a girl who was in a wheelchair with a degenerative nerve disease, Mia Lee was just too happy.

"I keep expecting more from the plotline than what's currently here," one publisher wrote. "What if it was about sisters who were twins, and one had Charcot-Marie-Tooth and one didn't? That would create a more important conflict." Another said that Mia Lee's character didn't seem suited for a lighthearted story. Finally, my agent told me, "I just don't think people are ready for this type of story for this type of character."

What she meant is that Mia Lee, my sassy, YouTube-loving heroine, differed too much from the convention of what a disabled kid is supposed to be like. There are very few stories about kids in wheelchairs, and there are even fewer with a disabled person who is cheerful and happy. Disability is always seen as a misfortune, and disabled characters are simply opportunities to demonstrate the kindness of the able-bodied protagonists.

For once, I want to see the disabled kids not in the hospital, but in the school cafeteria eating lunch with their friends. I wanted young readers to think of disabled kids not as miserable people to be pitied, but as people living normal lives in spite of their challenges. I want young readers to see disabled kids as *friends*, people to gossip with, to take selfies with and to go see movies with on the weekends. Not having books that show disability in a lighthearted way makes it harder for everyone else to see disability as a normal part of life.

Although I wasn't able to find a publisher who believed in that kind of story, I used the funds from my Kickstarter to self-publish the book on Amazon. "Mia Lee Is Wheeling Through Middle School" was released at the National Youth Transitions Center, and has sold hundreds of copies to parents and kids around the country.

Since its publication, I've gone back to being your average middle schooler. I was in my school play, and now I am getting ready to graduate. On the weekends, I go to the library, where sometimes, I see my book on the "just returned" shelf. I often wonder who had it checked out. Maybe it was someone who would go on to invite the special needs kid in his class over for a play date. Or maybe, it was another kid with a disability, who could point to the pages and say: "She's just like me! And she's happy, too!"

In My Chronic Illness, I Found a Deeper Meaning

ELLIOT KUKLA

I BECAME DISABLED OVERNIGHT IN A CAR ACCIDENT. THE CAR ACCIDENT was a dream, but the disability was real.

I dreamed I was driving through the ravaged streets of Oakland, California, at the end of the world. I turned the corner and careened inescapably into a white chemical blaze. I woke with a start, the white flash still burning behind my eyes, the worst headache of my life piercing my left temporal lobe. I remembered my mother having a brain aneurysm years before and knew the "worst headache of my life" was not to be ignored. My wife and I hurried to the hospital, expecting life to change forever. Once at the emergency room, things moved quickly: CT scans were ordered, crystal clear spinal fluid was drawn from my back. Eight hours later, I was told I was perfectly healthy.

What they meant, but wouldn't say, was that they didn't know what was wrong. Over the next weeks and months, it became obvious that I was far from well. The terrible headaches continued, I developed burning nerve pain all over my torso, I was wrapped in a thick brain fog, I sprouted mouth ulcers, I was crushed with exhaustion. I would open my mouth and be unable to speak. I could get lost in my own house between bedroom and bathroom, and forget my wife's name. I started having seizures.

By then, I had discovered that I was no longer trusted by my doctors about my own body or experiences. I reported odd, terrifying and sudden physical changes; they recommended cognitive behavioral therapy and Weight Watchers. I felt exiled from the world of the well, isolated by thick walls of suspicion. I'm used to feeling like an outsider; I'm the first openly transgender rabbi ordained by a mainstream movement (Reform Judaism). I am used to being rejected and told I should not exist. But nothing prepared me for the outsider status of being chronically ill.

Think about that for a moment: Approximately 0.6 percent of American adults identify as transgender, just under 0.2 percent of the world population is Jewish, and 100 percent of us will get sick, yet it is being chronically sick that makes me feel like an outsider. That's how much our society fears and rejects the core human experience of being ill, of having a body that gets sick, that ages, that is not controllable.

I went from doctor to doctor looking for answers, but overnight I had gone from being a trusted rabbi and chaplain (who works with seriously ill and dying people on hospital medical teams) to a "hysterical" chronically ill person. Though I had seen it happen to my clients, I now understood firsthand that being disbelieved is nearly universal for people with chronic illnesses, especially those that are largely invisible or hard to diagnose or both. I had believed that as a health care professional, equipped with skills and advocates to navigate the system, I would be treated differently. I soon learned how hubristic that was.

Eventually, because of the tireless advocacy of my wife, I was diagnosed with central nervous system lupus (an autoimmune disease that attacks the brain and central nervous system), as well as fibromyalgia, chronic fatigue syndrome and complex migraines. My lupus diagnosis would later be taken away and then given back countless times as suited the needs of health insurance and disability insurance companies to sort and manage me and decide how much care I was entitled to. The needs of my body were virtually irrelevant in this process as my diagnosis become a monetized affair where I had to jump through increasingly difficult hoops to "prove" it.

Like most of us, I had been raised to see illness as something temporary: a stopover on the way to recovery or to death, not a place to live. But weeks, months and then years passed, and I did not get better. My doctors, and even some friends and family members, suggested that I could get better if only I tried harder, relaxed more deeply, thought more positively. I became a lightning rod for others' fears of disability, dependence and fragility. In a political moment where health care is treated as a luxury and hurricane victims are blamed for their own disasters, an ethic of personal responsibility reigns. But sometimes, sick people just stay sick. And there's no meditation, medication, positive outlook, exercise or smoothie that can fix it.

Eventually, I stopped hoping to be well, or even pretending that I lived in that future-heavy land of hope anymore. I stopped trying to "overcome" my body and started living a present-tense life in chronic illness. As the pace of my life slowed, I could appreciate sensual pleasures in a new and heightened way: sunlight outside my bedroom window, my dog's velvety fur, a cool breeze in my garden, richly colored flowers. On days when my brain was too fogged to do anything, I let myself float in and out of a rich, infinitely layered dream world.

With great difficulty, I learned how to accept care. A child of neglectful and absent parents, I had been fiercely independent for most of my life; now, as fatigue gripped my body, I needed help preparing food, showering, doing laundry, managing my medications. This demanded a difficult, profoundly spiritual vulnerability. I realized that if I were truly to see myself as equal to my seriously ill clients, and not performing a kind of "charity" in my work, I had to come to terms with the necessity of interdependence.

We are born needing care and die needing care, and I am no exception. At brief moments in the middle of life, we hold the illusion of independence, but we are always driving on roads we did not build, eating foods we did not pick or raise. Allowing the illusion of my own independence to drop away unmasked a fundamental truth of being human.

Like many people, I had once measured my worth by my capacity to produce things and experiences: to be productive at work, share responsibilities at home, "show up" equally in my friendships and rack up achievements. Being sick has been a long, slow detox from capitalist culture and its mandate that we never rest. Slowly, I found a deeper value in relationship beyond reciprocity: an unconditional love and care based in justice, and a belief that all humans deserve relationship, regardless of whether we can offer anything measurable back. In these discoveries, I've been led by other sick and disabled people, whose value had always been apparent to me. Amid the brilliant diversity of power wheelchairs, service dogs, canes and ice packs, it's easy to see that we matter just as we are.

Eventually, my body did change. I am now able to stay awake longer, and my pain has receded to a dull throb. I can leave the house more; I can visit my clients and mentor my hospice volunteers, for which I am grateful. But I don't see myself as cured, nor do I imagine a cure will come. This is merely another chapter in the life of my body. If I'm lucky enough to get old, my body will change again. Because of my illnesses and family history, I'm more likely to develop dementia. As I age, my body and mind will surely become more disabled. I will lose cognitive and sensory capacities. My skin and muscles will sag and disintegrate. I will depend more and more on other people. I will not be able to control my bowels or my surroundings as tightly. I will lose teeth, hair and precious memories. This is not a tragedy. This is what it means to be human.

A Disabled Life Is a Life Worth Living

BEN MATTLIN

In midsummer 2016, I learned of the death of Laurie Hoirup, a prominent 60-year-old disability rights advocate in California. Laurie drowned in the Sacramento River after a July 4 celebration. She was well-loved and accomplished. She'd served as a chief deputy director of the State Council on Developmental Disabilities for five years and wrote books about living with a disability.

Laurie's sudden and tragic death was not directly caused by her SMA, but it is a stark reminder of the vulnerability of disabled lives. She was deboarding a pleasure boat when the ramp to the dock shifted. The weight of her motorized wheelchair—and the fact that she was strapped into it—pulled her down into the water too rapidly for rescue.

Laurie's death had extra significance for me, a 53-year-old husband and father of two, in part because we shared a diagnosis: spinal muscular atrophy.

SMA is a congenital and progressive neuromuscular weakness akin to muscular dystrophy. Until recently, half the babies born with it would die before their second birthdays. Their hearts and lungs became too weak to continue. Medical care and understanding have improved the odds somewhat.

I initially manifested symptoms at about 6 months. I was unable to sit up, and doctors promptly called me a "floppy baby." I never walked or stood on my own. At the time, SMA was all but unheard of and nearly impossible to diagnose. Now it's estimated to occur in one of every 6,000 to 10,000 births worldwide.

For people like us, simply enduring can feel like a tremendous victory. One bad cold, though, could spell our end. If our lungs fill with phlegm, we lack the muscle strength to cough them clear. Pneumonia is common. Some treatments help, but respiratory complications— and their impact on the heart—remain a constant threat.

It's not generally acceptable in my segment of the disability community to harp on our defenselessness. Rather, the idea is to assert core competencies, to distance ourselves from the Jerry's Kids' model and anything else remotely pitiful. We seek fair treatment, rightful access to everything in society—jobs, romantic prospects, and so on. Highlighting the downside of disabilities seems counterproductive and self-pitying.

But the truth is, to live with a disability is to know an abiding sense of fragility. That isn't always easy, but it's not necessarily all bad either.

I decided long ago that if I'm going to like myself, I have to like the disability that has contributed to who I am. Today, my encroaching decrepitude is frequently a source of emotional strength, a motivator to keep fighting, to exercise my full abilities in whatever way possible. Let's face it, people with disabilities are nothing if not first-class problem-solvers. We find all manner of devices to enable us to raise a fork, drive a car or van, go to the beach. I now control my electric wheelchair with my lips, because my hands no longer function. These very words are being written with a voice-recognition computer.

True, it is a hassle having to devise alternative methods for living a normal life. But when it works, Oh, how good it feels! How triumphant and liberating! I'm proud of my persistence and creative coping skills.

Of course at times I grow despondent. I fall into what I call "useless cripple syndrome." Most of my able-bodied contemporaries are at the pinnacle of their careers, and I'm just getting by. I shouldn't complain, I tell myself. Unemployment among disabled people is crushingly high.

Because of this, I feel positively driven to make good use of every day that I'm not stuck in bed with a respiratory infection or other ailment. Yes, that may make me an overachiever. I graduated cum laude from Harvard at 21. I became a financial journalist, and my essays have been featured in major publications, including this one. My second book will be published next year. I don't say all this to boast. The point is, I want to accomplish everything I can while I still have the ability. I may feel fine today, but I can't count on tomorrow—or even an hour from now. I've seen too many friends in the disability community perish too young.

Not long after the shock of Laurie's fatal accident, the news came of a 14-year-old Wisconsin girl with SMA, Jerika Bolen, who was planning to end her own life by refusing life-sustaining treatment. Just a few weeks ago, she did, and died. News reports said that Jerika was comforted by the promise of an afterlife in which she would be able to move freely and escape her persistent physical pain.

My reaction to this is strong and difficult to express. Growing up with a disability, I often became isolated. Feeling devalued by my peers, with no confidence in my future, I experienced intermittent but profound depression. One can take only so many surgeries, so many bodily betrayals, so much rejection, before wanting to give up. Even today, I can pivot from utter terror over an itch I can't scratch or a bite of food I can't quite swallow, to almost unbelievable joy if I manage to clear my throat unassisted or zoom my motorized wheelchair through a crowded street. As disabled people, we are endlessly buffeted by circumstances beyond our control.

I dare not judge Jerika Bolen. I don't know the entirety of her situation. But I do wish she had found the will to live. I'm saddened—as were many others with S.M.A, and some disability rights groups—to think others might grow so weary or apprehensive that they follow her example. I hope she received the same level of intervention any other suicidal 14-year-old would. I wish I could have told her about the psychological alchemy that can turn frustration into an internal fuel. If I'd had the chance I would have told her that society needs its disabled people, too.

The perseverance to live fully with a profound disability comes, I think, in part from honestly facing your own powerlessness and frailty, and recognizing how much worse things have been and could still be. This can instill a delight in the now. In living with a disability, you've already dealt with much of what other people fear most, and if you come out on the other side you are, by definition, a survivor. The resolve required, and begrudging acceptance of what you can't change, may bring a kind of wisdom.

I realize that external conditions can make all the difference. My family has given me unflagging support. My parents fought to get me integrated into regular schools, long before it was mandated, and insisted I could become anything I wanted when I grew up. Today, my family's financial backing allows me to hire the full-time aides I need to live a productive life. My wife provides for my personal maintenance whenever paid staff isn't available. Without all this, I would not be where I am today, but I'd like to think I'd find a way to survive.

Laurie Hoirup lived a full, active life. I wish I could have persuaded Jerika Bolen and others like her to keep striving to do the same, not to put her hopes and dreams into the idea of a heaven of unfettered athleticism. I wish I could have convinced her that she wasn't better off dead than disabled.

ABOUT THE CONTRIBUTORS

John Altmann is an independent scholar in philosophy and a regular contributor to the "Popular Culture and Philosophy" book series.

Todd Balf, a former senior editor at *Outside* magazine, whose writing has appeared in The New York Times Magazine, GQ, Runner's World and elsewhere, is the author of "The Last River, The Darkest Jungle and Major."

Jennifer Bartlett is a co-editor of "Beauty is a Verb: The New Poetry of Disability."

Sheila Black is the author of four poetry collections, most recently "Iron, Ardent." She is a co-editor of "Beauty is a Verb: The New Poetry of Disability" and "The Right Way to Be Crippled and Naked: The Fiction of Disability."

Sasha Blair-Goldensohn is a software engineer with Google Maps, and co-founder of the Elevator Action Group at Rise and Resist (www.riseandresist.org/eag). He lives in New York with his two children, Theo and Sophie.

Cheri A. Blauwet, an assistant professor at Harvard Medical School, is a seven-time Paralympic medalist and serves on the board of the United States Olympic Committee.

Joseph P. Carter has a PhD in philosophy from the University of Georgia.

Laurie Clements Lambeth is the author of "Veil and Burn," a book of poems, and is at work on a memoir. She teaches medical humanities courses at the University of Houston. Her lyric essay, "Going Downhill From Here," was named a Notable Essay in 2017's "Best American Essays."

Randi Davenport is the award-winning author of "The Boy Who Loved Tornadoes," a memoir, and "The End of Always," a novel. Her essays and short fiction have appeared in The New York Times, Washington Post, Ontario Review, Alaska Quarterly Review, HuffPost and many others.

Luticha Andre Doucette is a businesswoman, writer, philanthropist, proud cat mom and activist located in Rochester, N.Y. In her spare time she volunteers, is president of the board of a local nonprofit, is an avid reader and a competitive fencer.

Jane Eaton Hamilton is the Canadian author of nine books. They have twice won the CBC Literary Prize for fiction and have had Notables in BASS and BAE. Their work is upcoming in BAX 2020.

Anne Finger is a Fellow at the American Academy in Berlin. Her most recent book is a novel, "A Woman, in Bed."

Dr. Joseph J. Fins is the E. William Davis, Jr., M.D. Professor of Medical Ethics at Weill

Cornell Medical College and Solomon Center Distinguished Scholar in Medicine, Bioethics and the Law at Yale Law School. He is the author of "Rights Come to Mind: Brain Injury, Ethics, and the Struggle for Consciousness."

Shane Fistell is a sculptor and painter who has taken part in five award-winning documentaries on Tourette syndrome. He was born in Toronto, Ontario, where he now lives and works as an assistant karate instructor for children.

Paula Fitzgibbons is an award-winning writer based in Southern California, who usually focuses on parenting, chronic illness, surviving abuse and social justice. She has been published in The New York Times, New York Magazine and Today's Parent, among other publications.

Kenny Fries is the author of "In the Province of the Gods," which received the Creative Capital literature grant, "The History of My Shoes and the Evolution of Darwin's Theory," which received the Outstanding Book Award from the Gustavus Meyers Center for the Study of Bigotry and Human Rights, and "Body, Remember: A Memoir."

Rosemarie Garland-Thomson is a professor of English and bioethics at Emory University. Her work brings disability culture, ethics and justice to a broad range of institutions and communities.

Jenny Giering is a theater composer who has been sick for five years. She and her husband, writer Sean Barry, are currently working on a musical about their journey through her chronic illness called "What We Leave Behind."

Ona Gritz is the author of the memoir "On the Whole: A Story of Mothering and Disability," and the poetry collections "Geode" and "Border Songs: A Conversation in Poems," written with Daniel Simpson.

Elizabeth Guffey is the author of numerous books, including "Designing Disability: Symbols, Space, and Society." She is also founding editor of the academic journal Design and Culture and currently heads the MA in Modern and Contemporary Art, Criticism and Theory at the State University of New York, Purchase College.

Ariel Henley is a writer whose work focuses primarily on what it means to live with a noticeable facial difference. You can read her work at www.arielhenley.com.

Edward Hoagland is a nature and travel writer, and the author, most recently, of "In the Country of the Blind," a novel.

Alex Hubbard became a regular columnist for The Tennessean shortly after this essay was published in The New York Times. He is now the assistant opinion editor and columnist at The Tennessean and lives near Nashville.

Liz Jackson is the founder of The Disabled List, a disability design self-advocacy organization, and WITH, a fellowship that helps match creative disabled people with design studios and other organizations.

Creating at the intersection of art and science, artist and writer **Elizabeth Jameson** uses medical technology to depict the beauty and complexity of the imperfect body. She lectures internationally on art, disability identity and the power of narrative in reshaping the way illness and disability are viewed in society.

Cyndi Jones is the vicar of Atonement Lutheran Church, San Diego, in the Evangelical Lutheran Church in America. She was the publisher of Mainstream magazine from 1982 to 1998 and the director of the Center for an Accessible Society from 1998 to 2010. (The author is not associated with any online version of Mainstream magazine.)

Anne Kaier's essay "Maple Lane" was mentioned on the list of Notables in the 2014 edition of "Best American Essays." Her memoir, "Home with Henry," is out from PS Books. Other work has appeared in The New York Times, Under the Sun, 1966, Gettysburg Review, Alaska Quarterly Review and Kenyon Review.

Georgina Kleege teaches disability studies and creative writing in the English Department at the University of California, Berkeley. Her most recent book is "More Than Meets the Eye: What Blindness Brings to Art."

Rachel Kolb is a writer and a PhD candidate in English literature at Emory University, where her work uses deafness and disability to shed light on broader American cultural ideas about the senses, language and communication. She was previously a Rhodes scholar at Oxford University.

Catherine Kudlick is a professor of history and the director of the Paul K. Longmore Institute on Disability at San Francisco State University. She is at work on a memoir about her experiences at the Colorado Center for the Blind.

Elliot Kukla is a rabbi at the Bay Area Jewish Healing Center where he provides spiritual care to those who are ill, dying or bereaved. He lives in Oakland with his wife, their kid and a menagerie of pets.

Emily Ladau is a passionate disability rights activist, writer, speaker, editor, podcaster and digital communications consultant whose work can be found on WordsIWheelBy.com. Emily's activism is driven by her firm belief that if we want the world to be accessible to people with all types of disabilities, we must make ideas and concepts surrounding disability accessible to the world.

Alaina Leary is an editor and a social media strategist at We Need Diverse Books. She lives with her wife, their two cats and lots of glitter.

Riva Lehrer is an artist, curator and writer whose portrait work was recently acquired by the National Portrait Gallery of the Smithsonian Museum. Her memoir, "Golem Girl," will be published by the One World imprint of Penguin Random House in spring 2020.

Gila Lyons's writing about mental health has appeared in The New York Times, O, The Oprah Magazine, Vice, Cosmopolitan, Salon, Health, Healthline, Ploughshares and other publications. She holds an MFA in literary nonfiction from Columbia University, and is at work on a memoir about seeking a natural cure for anxiety and panic disorder but falling prey to the underbelly of the alternative health movement. You can read more about her work at www.gilalyons.com.

Ben Mattlin is a freelance journalist and the author of "Miracle Boy Grows Up" and "In Sickness and in Health." In addition to The New York Times, he has written for the Washington Post, Los Angeles Times, Chicago Tribune, USA Today and NPR's "Morning Edition."

Molly McCully Brown is the author of "The Virginia State Colony For Epileptics and Feebleminded," and winner of the 2016 Lexi Rudnitsky First Book Prize. She teaches at Kenyon College, where she is a Kenyon Review Fellow.

Zack McDermott is the author of the forthcoming, "Gorilla and the Bird: A Memoir of Madness and a Mother's Love."

Catherine Monahon is a creative writer, editor and copywriter with a background in fine art. She works collaboratively with creative teams to tell stories that matter.

Jonathan Mooney is the author of "Learning Outside the Lines" and "The Short Bus: A Journey Beyond Normal." He is a co-founder of Eye to Eye, a national advocacy organization for people with learning differences.

Susannah Nevison is the author of poetry collections "Lethal Theater" and "Teratology." With Molly McCully Brown, she is the co-author of the forthcoming collaborative poetry collection, "In the Field Between Us." She teaches at Sweet Briar College.

JoAnna Novak is the author of the novel "I Must Have You" and the book-length poem "Noirmania." She is a founding editor of Tammy, a literary journal and chapbook press.

Valerie Piro is a doctoral student at Princeton University, where she studies early medieval social history. Her work on disability has been featured in Inside Higher Ed and the Harvard Law Record. She blogs about her life with paralysis at themightyval.com.

Emily Rapp Black is the author of "Poster Child: A Memoir" and "The Still Point of the Turning World," and is an assistant professor of creative writing at the University of California, Riverside.

Oliver Sacks (1933-2015) was a neurologist and a frequent contributor to The New York Times and other publications. "Mishearings," first published by the Times in 2015, is also included in his book "The River of Consciousness." His most recent book is "Everything in Its Place."

Katie Savin is a PhD candidate in Social Welfare at UC Berkeley, where she researches disability, poverty and the welfare state. A longtime proud, disabled public transit rider, she enjoys talking to strangers, teaching social welfare policy and writing.

Melissa Shang, born with a form of muscular dystrophy called Charcot-Marie-Tooth, is a 15-year-old disability activist who goes to Newton South High School. In 2014, Melissa launched a viral petition of a disabled American Girl doll that was featured in Cosmopolitan, USA Today, CBS, HLN, IB Times and other major news outlets and raised massive public attention to disability representation in children's toys. Currently, Melissa has published her first book, "Mia Lee is Wheeling Through Middle School."

Alice Sheppard is an award-winning disabled dancer and choreographer. She is the artistic director for Kinetic Light, a collaborative with Laurel Lawson and Michael Maag.

Daniel Simpson is the author of "School for the Blind," a collection of poems, and the blog Inside the Invisible. His book "Border Songs: A Conversation in Poems," written with Ona Gritz, was published by Finishing Line Press.

Brad Snyder is currently an adjunct professor of leadership at the United States Naval Academy and serves on the United States Olympic Committee board of directors. He is a five-time Paralympic gold medalist and is training to earn a spot on Team USA's roster for Tokyo.

Andrew Solomon is the author of "The Noonday Demon: An Atlas of Depression" and "Far From the Tree: Parents, Children and the Search for Identity."

Rivers Solomon is at work on her second novel.

Carol R. Steinberg is a lawyer, writer, speaker, accessibility consultant and disability activist in Boston. Her writing has appeared in the Boston Globe, Huffington Post, The New York Times and elsewhere.

Jillian Weise is the author of "The Amputee's Guide to Sex," "The Colony," "The Book of Goodbyes" and "Cyborg Detective." She created the web series Tips for Writers by Tipsy Tullivan and performs as Tipsy across social media.

Abby L. Wilkerson is an associate professor of writing at George Washington University and the author of "Diagnosis: Difference—The Moral Authority of Medicine."

Alice Wong is a media maker, research consultant and disability activist based in San Francisco. She is the founder and director of the Disability Visibility Project, an online community dedicated to creating, sharing and amplifying disability media and culture.